Depersonalization: A New Look at a Neglected Syndrome

Depersonalization: A New Look at a Neglected Syndrome

Mauricio Sierra, M.D., Ph.D.

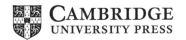

CAMBRIDGE
UNIVERSITY PRESS

CAMBRIDGE UNIVERSITY PRESS
Cambridge, New York, Melbourne, Madrid, Cape Town,
Singapore, São Paulo, Delhi, Tokyo, Mexico City

Cambridge University Press
The Edinburgh Building, Cambridge CB2 8RU, UK

Published in the United States of America by
Cambridge University Press, New York

www.cambridge.org
Information on this title: www.cambridge.org/9780521874984

First published 2009
Reprinted 2010

A catalogue record for this publication is available from the British Library

Library of Congress Cataloguing in Publication data

ISBN 978-0-521-87498-4 Hardback

To Gloria, in gratitude for the gift of love

Contents

Acknowledgements

It would be impossible to name all the people who in one way or another have made this work possible. Some of them, however, deserve a special mention. A heartfelt 'thank you' goes out to them:

To Ricardo Jose Toro who in the early days of my training in psychiatry fostered my interest in dissociation and allowed my mind to run free.

To German Berrios, a most inspiring teacher, scholar and free-spirited mind.

To Anthony David for his support, trust and inextinguishable drive along the years. Thanks to him the first Depersonalization Disorder Clinic in Europe became a tangible and successful reality.

To the Pilkington trusts, and in particular to Philip and Gloria Pilkington, whose enthusiasm and support has been a real force behind the curtains.

To all the patients, who generously have contributed to turn their suffering into knowledge.

Introduction

Depersonalization is a fascinating and intriguing phenomenon which becomes, for those who experience it, a significant source of distress and alienation, and poses a direct challenge to long-held, unquestioned assumptions regarding their existence and identity. Indeed, the person affected with depersonalization 'complains spontaneously that his or her mental activity, body and surroundings are changed in their quality, so as to be unreal, remote or automatized. Among the varied phenomena of the syndrome, patients complain most frequently of loss of emotions and feelings of estrangement or detachment from their thinking, their body or the real world. In spite of the dramatic nature of the experience, the patient is aware of the unreality of the change. The sensorium is normal and the capacity for emotional expression intact' (World Health Organization, 1992).

Since the condition was first described (half a century before it was named), during the first half of the nineteenth century, depersonalization has been found to be commonplace in psychiatric patients. For example, Schilder (1935), who wrote extensively on depersonalization believed it to be present, at some stage, in 'almost every neurosis'. A similar view led a panel of clinicians to conclude that, after anxiety and depression, depersonalization was the most frequent symptom seen in psychiatry (Stewart, 1964), while others emphasized its frequent occurrence in association with neurological conditions (Brock and Wiesel, 1942). Such ubiquitous nature led early writers to believe that depersonalization must be related to functions relevant to the understanding of both normal and abnormal mentation: "the syndrome is related to so many urgent questions of medical and normal psychology that it is worth studying in a large number of patients" (Mayer-Gross, 1935). Coinciding with the rise of interest in the study of altered mental states of consciousness during the 1960s and 1970s, there was a significant increase in the number of publications dealing with theoretical, philosophical as well as empirical research on depersonalization. It became well established for example, that fleeting experiences of depersonalization were commonplace among teenagers, as well as in people facing life-threatening situations. In turn, empirical studies on large samples of patients confirmed the view that depersonalization was indeed highly prevalent among psychiatric in-patients, as well as in patients with depression, anxiety disorders and schizophrenia (Brauer *et al.*, 1970; Hunter *et al.*, 2004). However, unlike the case with equally ubiquitous symptoms such as anxiety and depressed mood, the high prevalence of depersonalization was taken to mean that it was so non-specific as to lack any clinical relevance. A profusion of literature emphasizing depersonalization in its non-specific guise, seems to have had the effect of eclipsing clinical observations, which suggested that, just as it was the case with depression or anxiety, depersonalization did become, in some cases, a chronic, distressing and incapacitating condition in its own right (Shorvon, 1946). Roth (1959, p. 587) criticized this neglecting bias with unusual clarity:

It is traditional to begin papers such as this dealing with depersonalization by paying tribute to the ubiquity and versatility of the phenomenon citing in illustration the experiences of Wordsworth, Amiel and Charles Morgan and continuing with depersonalization occurring in schizophrenia, affective disorder, obsessional states, temporal lobe epilepsy, head injury, encephalitis, carbon monoxide poisoning, hashish intoxication, and botulism....such a list is somewhat misleading ... as it appears to confer an equal status to the very rare and the common place. And a similar one could be compiled for the majority of entities known to psychiatry.

The existence of severe, chronic clinical presentations of depersonalization had been clearly described since the early nineteenth century, but became particularly well established in 1946 with the publication of an impressive series of 66 patients suffering with a distinct form of chronic depersonalization that could not be attributed to any other mental pathology (Shorvon, 1946). Two decades later similar cases were again well documented by Roth (1959), who in addition to the chronic nature of depersonalization, drew attention to the concomitant severe distress and anxiety experienced by those affected. Unfortunately, such observations suggesting a chronic and disabling form of depersonalization have traditionally been met with disbelief within mainstream psychiatry. A comment found in a fairly recent publication illustrates well this commonly held view: 'Despite a lack of convincing empirical justification, the DSM-IV and the ICD-10 contain depersonalization as a separate disorder' (Parnas and Handest, 2003).

In the last decade, however, there has been a renewed interest in the study of chronic, pathological forms of depersonalization not explainable by any other mental illness. Two large independent series of cases on both sides of the Atlantic have been systematically assessed and found to converge on clinical features, demographics and course of illness (Simeon *et al.*, 2003; Baker *et al.*, 2003). It is now known that this form of depersonalization (referred to as Depersonalization Disorder by the DSM-IV, or as Depersonalization–Derealization syndrome by the ICD-10) typically begins during mid to late teens, and tends to run a continuous, unremitting course for years and even decades (Simeon, 2004). Unfortunately, the condition has been shown refractory to most conventional medications used in psychiatry, and at the time of writing there is no officially recognized treatment (Sierra, 2008). The quality and strength of the data published by three independent clinical research centres are such that the existence of a primary form of chronic depersonalization can be safely established as a clinical fact. This is indeed reflected on current official classifications, although the prevailing view is that the condition is exceptionally rare. Such a view is, for example, still enshrined in the ICD-10 definition of 'depersonalization–derealization syndrome', which qualifies it as being 'very rare'. How does this view square with current epidemiological data? A few studies in the general population have now been carried out which suggest that the prevalence of chronic, pathological depersonalization lies around 1% (Hunter et al., 2004; Johnson et al., 2006; Michal et al., 2009). In other words, such findings would seem to suggest that depersonalization disorder is as prevalent as other well-known mainstream psychiatric conditions such as schizophrenia or manic-depressive illness. If that is the case, however, how is it that most clinicians believe it to be so rare? There may be several reasons for this: most psychiatrists are still trained to believe that depersonalization disorder is extremely rare or non-existent, and that, when present, it is usually a secondary, almost irrelevant symptom of another condition such as depression. Not surprisingly, this leads to a high rate of misdiagnosis. In fact, it is known that, from the moment patients make initial contact with a mental health service, it usually takes up to 12 years until the right diagnosis is made (Hunter et al., 2003). Underdiagnosis may also stem from the fact that patients are often reluctant to divulge their symptoms out of fears of being thought mad by others or due to difficulties in describing such an ineffable experience (Simeon, 2004). In this regard, failure to ask screening questions during assessment interviews is also a known element contributing to non-detection (Edwards and Angus, 1972).

The above scenario would not be unknown in the recent history of psychiatry. For example, up until the early 1980s, the prevailing view was that obsessive compulsive disorder (OCD) was an extremely rare condition, with a prevalence not higher than 0.05% in the general population. However, the Epidemiology Catchment Area survey, and subsequent epidemiological studies across the world showed the prevalence to be 50 to 100 times more common than previously thought, being in fact 'twice as common as schizophrenia or panic disorder' (Rasmussen and Eisen, 1990; Weissman et al., 1994).

The last decade has seen an unprecedented resurgence in research on depersonalization. It is indeed no exaggeration to say that, as a result of the establishment of specialised clinics and research programmes both in the US and in Europe, more has been learned about the condition in the last 10 years than in the previous 100 years. The availability of large samples of patients meeting strict criteria for depersonalization disorder has afforded a unique opportunity to carry out systematic research on the phenomenology, and clinical features of the condition. In fact, systematic descriptions of large series of patients with depersonalization disorder have shown striking clinical overlaps in regards to the different symptom domains that characterize the condition (Sierra *et al.*, 2005; Simeon *et al.*, 2008). A similar convergence has also been found between modern and historical cases, suggesting a degree of clinical homogeneity seldom encountered in clinical psychiatry. It is now clear that, rather than being restricted to the experience of 'unreality feelings', depersonalization is a complex phenomenon characterized by several symptom domains of which 'derealization' is only one (Sierra *et al.*, 2005; Simeon *et al.*, 2008). On a clinical level, it is also becoming clear that, in addition to its chronic, incapacitating variety (i.e. depersonalization disorder), the presence of depersonalization in patients with other primary diagnoses may have clinical and prognostic implications. It has been shown, for example, that its presence in patients with panic disorder or depression constitutes a marker of severity, and its presence in depression seems associated with poorer response to treatment (Mula *et al.*, 2007).

The emerging view places depersonalization along a spectrum of severity, which goes from the fleeting and seemingly benign depersonalization experiences of youth, moving on to depersonalization as a comorbid manifestation of other psychiatric conditions, and finally to severe, disabling cases of constant depersonalization which cannot be accounted for by any other psychiatric condition. Interestingly, patients often show a dynamic longitudinal progression of severity along the continuum. Thus, it is not rare to find patients who having experienced fleeting depersonalization experiences in their childhood and early teens, go on to develop severe depersonalization in the context of depression or an anxiety disorder, which after responding to treatment, leave depersonalization as a sole, unchallenged condition for years (Baker *et al.*, 2003). This dimensional view of depersonalization brings coherence to what used to be a set of scattered, seemingly unrelated observations. For example, it has now been shown that experiences of emotional abuse in childhood predispose to the occurrence of depersonalization in both its pathological and nonclinical forms (Simeon *et al.*, 2001; Michal *et al.*, 2007).

Recent research using psychophysiological as well as functional neuroimaging approaches are revealing distinct abnormalities, which supports the idea that the condition is firmly grounded on neurobiological mechanisms (Phillips and Sierra, 2003). The significance of such objective findings is particularly relevant for a condition like depersonalization, the clinical manifestations of which are entirely subjective, and mostly confined to the experiential domain of self-awareness.

The main purpose for writing this book has been to pull together all the different research threads of the last decade, and to relate them to the larger canvas of more than 100 years of research and thinking into this enigmatic condition.

REFERENCES

Baker, D., Hunter, E., Lawrence, E. *et al.* (2003). Depersonalisation disorder: clinical features of 204 cases. *British Journal of Psychiatry*, **182**, 428–433.

Brauer, R., Harrow, M., Tucker, G. J. (1970). Depersonalization phenomena in psychiatric patients. *British Journal of Psychiatry*, **117**, 509–515.

Brock, S., Wiesel, B. (1942). Derealization and depersonalization: their occurrence in organic and psychogenic states. *Diseases of the Nervous System*, **3**, 139–149.

Edwards, J. G., Angus, J. W. (1972). Depersonalization. *British Journal of Psychiatry*, **120**, 242–244.

Hunter, E. C., Phillips, M. L., Chalder, T., Sierra, M., David, A. S. (2003). Depersonalisation disorder: a cognitive-behavioural conceptualisation. *Behaviour Research and Therapy*, **41**, 1451–1467.

Hunter, E. C., Sierra, M., David, A. S. (2004). The epidemiology of depersonalisation and derealisation. A systematic review. *Social Psychiatry and Psychiatric Epidemiology*, **39**, 9–18.

Johnson, J. G., Cohen, P., Kasen, S., Brook, J. S. (2006). Dissociative disorders among adults in the community, impaired functioning, and axis I and II comorbidity. *Journal of Psychiatry Research*, **40**, 131–140.

Mayer-Gross, W. (1935). On depersonalisation. *British Journal of Medical Psychology*, **15**, 103–122.

Michal, M., Beutel, M. E., Jordan, J., Zimmermann, M., Wolters, S., Heidenreich, T. (2007). Depersonalization, mindfulness, and childhood trauma. *Journal of Nervous and Mental Disease*, **195**, 693–696.

Michal, M., Wiltink, J., Subic-Wrana, C. *et al.* (2009). Prevalence, correlates and predictors of depersonalization experiences in the German general population. *Journal of Nervous and Mental Disease*, in press.

Mula, M., Pini, S., Cassano, G. B. (2007). The neurobiology and clinical significance of depersonalization in mood and anxiety disorders: a critical reappraisal. *Journal of Affective Disorders*, **99**, 91–99.

Parnas, J., Handest, P. (2003). Phenomenology of anomalous self-experience in early schizophrenia. *Comprehensive Psychiatry*, **44**, 121–134.

Phillips, M.L., Sierra, M. (2003). Depersonalization disorder: a functional neuroanatomical perspective. *Stress*, **6**, 157–165.

Rasmussen, S. A., Eisen, J. L. (1990). Epidemiology of obsessive compulsive disorder. *Journal of Clinical Psychiatry*, **51** Suppl, 10–13.

Roth, M. (1959). The phobic anxiety-depersonalisation syndrome. *Proceedings of the Royal Society of Medicine*, **52**, 587–595.

Schilder, P. (1935). *The Image and Appearance of the Human Body*. London: Kegan Paul.

Shorvon, H. J. (1946). The depersonalisation syndrome. *Proceedings of the Royal Society of Medicine*, **39**, 779–792.

Sierra, M. (2008). Depersonalization disorder: pharmacological approaches. *Expert Review of Neurotherapeutics*, **8**, 19–26.

Sierra, M., Baker, D., Medford, N., David, A. S. (2005). Unpacking the depersonalization syndrome: an exploratory factor analysis on the Cambridge Depersonalization Scale. *Psychological Medicine*, **35**, 1523–1532.

Simeon, D. (2004). Depersonalisation disorder: a contemporary overview. *CNS Drugs*, **18**, 343–354.

Simeon, D., Guralnik, O., Schmeidler, J., Sirof, B., Knutelska, M. (2001). The role of childhood interpersonal trauma in depersonalization disorder. *American Journal of Psychiatry*, **158**, 1027–1033.

Simeon, D., Knutelska, M., Nelson, D., Guralnik, O. (2003). Feeling unreal: a depersonalization disorder update of 117 cases. *Journal of Clinical Psychiatry*, **64**, 990–997.

Simeon, D., Kozin, D. S., Segal, K., Lerch, B., Dujour, R., Giesbrecht, T. (2008). De-constructing depersonalization: further evidence for symptom clusters. *Psychiatry Research*, **157**, 303–306.

Stewart, W. A. (1964). Panel on depersonalization. *Journal of the American Psychoanalytic Association*, **12**, 171–186.

Weissman, M. M., Bland, R. C., Canino, G. J. *et al.* (1994). The cross national epidemiology of obsessive compulsive disorder. The Cross National Collaborative Group. *Journal of Clinical Psychiatry*, **55** Suppl, 5–10.

World Health Organization (1992). F48.1. Depersonalisation–derealisation syndrome. In *The ICD-10 Classification of Mental and Behavioural Disorders*. Clinical descriptions and diagnostic guidelines. Geneva: World Health Organization. pp. 171–173.

1

A history of depersonalization

Introduction

The term and concept depersonalization appeared during the late nineteenth century to name a cluster of apparently related experiences usually described as ineffable feelings of disembodiment, loss of feelings and a sense of unreality regarding the self and surroundings. During the early part of the twentieth century, the term derealization was introduced to refer to the latter aspect of depersonalization but it has since been reified into another concept. Depersonalization is currently defined in DSM-IV as: "an alteration in the perception or experience of the self so that one feels detached from, and as if one is an outside observer of", one's "mental processes or body (e.g. feeling like one is in a dream)" and derealization as "an alteration in the perception or experience of the external world so that it seems strange or unreal (e.g. people may seem unfamiliar or mechanical)" (American Psychiatric Association, 1994).

This chapter will trace the history of depersonalization as it gradually evolved from early scattered descriptions, their subsequent convergence under the new term 'depersonalization' at the end of the nineteenth century, and the ensuing attempts to understand and relate the condition to the landscape of 'mental faculties' known at the time. A historical understanding of how depersonalization came to be construed would in itself constitute a good introduction to the condition, as all its nuances are still as relevant today as they were a century ago (Sierra and Berrios, 1997).

Early historical descriptions

Early descriptions of experiences redolent of 'depersonalization' can be found in the medical literature since the early nineteenth century. For example, as early as 1845, Griesinger quoted a letter written by a patient to Esquirol, the prominent French psychiatrist:

I continue to suffer constantly; I don't have a moment of comfort, nor experience human sensations. Even though I am surrounded by all that can render life happy and agreeable, in me the faculty of enjoyment and sensation is wanting or have become physical impossibilities. In everything, even in the most tender caresses of my children, I find only bitterness, I cover them with kisses, but there is something between their lips and mine; and this horrid something is between me and the enjoyments of life. My existence is incomplete. The functions and acts of ordinary life, it is true, still remain to me; but in every one of them there is something lacking. That is, the sensation which is proper to them ... Each of my senses, each part of my proper self is as if it were separated from me and can no longer afford me any sensation. This impossibility seems to depend upon a void which I feel in the front of my head and to be due to a diminished sensibility over my whole body, for it seems to me that I never actually reach the objects that I touch. I no longer experience the internal feeling of the air when I breath ... My eyes see and my spirit perceives, but the sensation of what I see is completely absent (Griesinger, 1845, p. 157).

Griesinger seemed well aquainted with such descriptions as he had commented earlier:

We sometimes hear the insane, especially melancholics, complain of a quite different kind of anaesthesia ... I see, I hear, I feel, they say but the object does not reach me; I cannot receive the sensation; It seems to me as if there was a wall between me and the external world' (my italics) p. 67.

However, rather than just being an accompanying symptom of depression, Griesinger seemed aware that at times such symptoms seemed to lead an independent course: '*This very remarkable state, which the patients themselves have much difficulty in describing, and which we also have ourselves observed in several cases as the predominant and most lasting symptom ...*' (Griesinger, 1845; my italics p. 157).

In a similar way, Zeller (1838) reported five patients, all of whom "*complained almost in the same terms of a lack of sensations ... to them it was a total lack of feelings, as if they were dead ... they claimed they could think clearly, and properly about everything, but the essential was lacking even in their thoughts ... A criminal is better off in that he dreads the scaffold. At least he can experience fear of death and they might envy him for that*" (my italics), pp. 524–525.

At around the same period, in France, Esquirol (1838) described similar experiences in patients: "*An abyss, they say, separates them from the external world, I hear, I see, I touch, say many lypemaniacs, but I am not as I formerly was. Objects do not come to me, they do not identify themselves with my being; a thick cloud, a veil changes the hue and aspect of objects*" (p. 414). Another great French psychiatrist, Billod (1847) described a patient who complained of similar experiences: "*she claimed to feel as if she were not dead or alive, as if living in a continuous dream ... objects [in her environment] looked as if surrounded by a cloud; people seemed to move like shadows, and words seemed to come from a far away world*" (p. 187).

The first systematic account of such experiences was provided by Maurice Krishaber (1873), a Hungarian ENT specialist working in France who, under the category 'Névropathie Cérébro-Cardiaque' reported 38 patients showing a mixture of anxiety, fatigue and depressive mood. Krishaber noted that over one-third of these patients complained of a baffling and distressing mental experience, characterized by the loss of a feeling of reality. He went on to suggest that these phenomena resulted from sensory dysfunction (see below).

The construction of depersonalization

It was the psychologist Ludovic Dugas who first introduced the word depersonalization into the psychiatric literature. Dugas (1894) first came across 'depersonalization' whilst exploring the psychopathology of déjà-vu and related experiences, which at the time were designated by the generic name of 'false memories'. Thus, Dugas wrote: *"In 1894, when dealing with false memories, I had not yet knowledge of depersonalization. Not realising its novelty, I missed [the phenomenon] when I first met it"* (1898a) p. 424. Soon enough, however, Dugas published a series of papers on the subject (1898b, 1912, 1915, 1936) and wrote a monograph entitled *La Dépersonnalisation*, which he co-authored with the French neurologist Maurice Moutier (Dugas and Moutier, 1911).

Dugas defined depersonalization as "A state in which there is the feeling or sensation that thoughts and acts elude the self (*le moi sent ses pensées et ses actes lui échapper*) and become strange (*lui devenir étranger*); there is an alienation of personality (during the nineteenth century the term personality referred mainly to the subjective experience of self); in other words a depersonalization" (Dugas and Moutier, 1911, p. 13). In fact, he thought of the condition as resulting from a dysfunction of a putative mental faculty, which Dugas termed 'personalization', whose function was to 'personalize' mental events: "Personalization is the act of psychical synthesis, of appropriation or attribution of states to the self" (Dugas and Moutier, 1911).

Dugas acknowledged that he had taken the term depersonalization from an intriguing paragraph found in H. F. Amiel's *Journal Intime*. The Swiss philosopher (1821–1881) had written in his personal diary: "All is strange to me; I am, as it were, outside my own body and individuality; I am *depersonalised*, detached, cut adrift." (Amiel, 1933; p. 275). This seems to have been interpreted by Dugas as a literal description of Amiel's mental experiences. However, contextualized reading makes it unclear to what extent his descriptions of alienation were metaphorical rather than full-blown depersonalization experiences. For example, a few paragraphs later, Amiel clarifies: "It seems to me that my mental transformations are but *Philosophical experiences*." (my italics) p. 275.

Early theories of depersonalization

The sensory theory

One of the earliest views of depersonalization stemmed from a literal interpretation of those depersonalization complaints, which suggested a sensory distortion. One of the earliest writers to suggest that feelings of unreality might stem from pathological changes in the sensory apparatus was Krishaber himself. He believed that "multiple sensory distortions led to experiences of self-strangeness" (Krishaber, 1873, p. 171).

In his *Les maladies de la Personnalité*, Ribot (1895) endorsed a sensory dysfunction view and reported patients (some taken from Krishaber) who seem to describe anomalous body experiences 'of being separated from the universe, of feeling their bodies as if wrapped with an isolating substance interposing between themselves and the external world' (Ribot, 1895, p. 106). According to Ribot such experiences were caused by 'physiological abnormalities whose immediate effect is to produce a change in coenesthesia' (Ribot, 1895, pp. 105–106). The latter term commonly referred to a general sense of bodily existence, not reducible to any of the known sensory modalities (Berrios, 1981; Schiller, 1984). In the same vein, Séglas indicated that *"troubles de la perception personnelle des sensations internes, cénesthétiques"* might underlie typical depersonalization feelings. He described, for example, the case of a female patient with agoraphobia who 'lost awareness of body' every time she walked down the road: "it seems to me as if I am split into two, I lose the awareness of my body, which feels as if it is in front of me, I walk, and I am aware of it but I do not have awareness of my own identity, that it is actually me who is walking" (Séglas, 1895, p. 131). In a similar guise, Sollier brought attention to complaints of disturbing and baffling sensations in the head, which he ascribed to loss of 'cerebral coenesthesia' (Sollier, 1907, 1910). The conceptual roots of such 'sensory hypotheses' can be traced to eighteenth century beliefs on an association between bodily sensations and the 'feeling of the self'. For example, Lamarck (1820, p. 191) wrote: "it is an internal sensation, a very obscure feeling, that provides the individual with his consciousness of being".

In German-speaking psychiatry, Wernicke conceived of body awareness (*Psomatopsyche*) as related to muscle proprioceptive sensations (*Muskelsinn*). *Somatopsychosen*, according to Wernicke, were disorders characterized by distortions of body awareness such as Cotard's syndrome and depersonalization. One of his patients complained: "that her body had become stiff, and that she had to keep touching herself to feel the heaviness of her body. She felt as if it was dead and numb, as if it was bereft of circulation, even though she could feel her pulse and the beats of her heart. Such feelings also involved her sensory organs: she could hear, but felt that her eyes were fixed to her head, and couldn't move them" (Wernicke, 1906, p. 242). This hypothesis was developed further by Foerster (one of Wernicke's disciples), who suggested that all sensations were composed of: (a) a specific sensory component, i.e. visual, auditory, etc. and (b) a concomitant muscular sensation arising from the movement itself and which served to guide the sensory apparatus to the stimulus. In healthy individuals, subjective feelings of reality and vividness resulted from a synchronic action of these two components; in depersonalized patients, the proprioceptive component failed to reach consciousness (Foerster, 1903).

A similar view was defended by Pick, who in his article 'Disorders of the awareness of the self' (*Pathologie des Ich-Bewusstseins*) suggested that depersonalization was accompanied by a disturbance of sensory perception (*Störungen der Sinnesperception*) which, he hoped, might one day be confirmed by new research techniques (Pick, 1909).

The sensory hypothesis was challenged by Dugas and Moutier (1911), who suggested that, by taking too literally their patients' complaints, Krishaber (1873) and Taine (1906) had been misled into believing that they were suffering from some form of sensory pathology. Dugas and Moutier argued instead that such talk reflected metaphorical descriptions of experiences difficult to articulate in words. Thus they criticized Taine (1906) for not realizing that Krishaber's case No38 (1973) was speaking in a *'style métaphorique'* (Dugas and Moutier, 1911, p. 22).

Pierre Janet (1928) also rejected the sensory hypothesis of depersonalization by means of counter-examples. Thus, he reported patients who, in spite of having clear sensory pathology (such as the diplopia and loss of joint sense caused by neurosyphilis), did not complain of sensations of unreality (*sentiment de l'irréel*). Likewise, he also argued that many patients suffering from depersonalization were, in fact, normal from the sensory viewpoint (Janet, 1928, p. 89).

Theories based on faculty psychology

The view that the mind was constituted by faculties or modules, more or less independent in their functioning, came into early nineteenth-century European psychopathology from Kant and the Scottish philosophers of Common Sense (Hilgard, 1980). In France, it arrived via Laromiguière, Cousin, Royer-Collard, Garnier and the phrenological movement (Berrios, 1996). Faculty psychology was crucial to the development of theories of brain localization, psychiatric classification and typologies of character and personality. Soon, nineteenth-century alienists asked (e.g. Esquirol) what disorders might arise if the faculties of the mind became independently diseased. This nosological approach was still predominant at the time that Dugas started to explore the phenomenology and mechanisms of depersonalization (Sierra and Berrios, 1996). The implicit assumption was that depersonalization must be reducible to a dysfunctional manifestation of one of the known 'mental faculties'. There was, however, no agreement as to which 'faculty' this was. Although Dugas and Moutier (1911) had already made reference to 'personalization' as a putative 'synthetic' mental function, whose function was impaired in depersonalization, most subsequent writers attempted to link depersonalization to more basic and better established 'mental faculties' (Sierra and Berrios, 1997).

Memory

The view that depersonalization might be seen as a manifestation of a memory impairment, referred to a specific nineteenth-century idea, which conceived of a number of mental states, characterized by ineffable, unjustified anomalous feelings of familiarity in response to a particular situation (e.g. déjà vu), as reflecting dysfunctional 'remembering'. In short, whilst some writers had conceived these phenomena in terms of a perceptual anomaly, others such as Sander, Pick and Kraepelin proposed the view that they arose from qualitative disturbances of memory referred to as 'paramnesias' (Marková and Berrios, 2000).

In *Über Erinnerungfälschungen* (on memory falsifications), Kraepelin (1887) endorsed such a view, and went on to describe what seemed like personal brushes with depersonalization (e.g. "according to my experience", "in my own experience"): "At that moment it seems to us that all of a sudden the surroundings become hazy, as something quite remote and of no concern at all ... The impressions from the surroundings do not convey the familiar picture of everyday reality, instead they become dream-like or shadowy... as if seen through a veil" (p. 410). During the episode there can be 'a feeling of complete thought-emptiness' (p. 411). For Kraepelin, these feelings of unreality (not yet known as 'depersonalization') were part of the 'déjà vu' experience (then not yet named thus), and therefore resulting from a putative memory disturbance.

Seven years later, Dugas reported a case with concurrent depersonalization and 'déjà vu' experiences (Dugas, 1894), although – as mentioned above – he did not notice (or believe) at the time that they were separate clinical phenomena (Dugas, 1898a,b). Indeed, in that early paper, Dugas regarded the presence of depersonalization as evidence for the view that 'déjà vu' was a form of 'double consciousness' (*dédoublement de la personnalité*): "I would say that false memory is a special case of double personality ... [in which] the subject experiencing a false memory is [actually] aware of his becoming another" (1894, p. 43). He quoted a patient as saying: "I heard my voice as if I had heard the voice of a stranger, but at the same time I recognised it as mine; I knew it was me talking, but I was speaking as if it was old and remote".

Four years later, Dugas (1898a,b) reported the phenomenon under a new name (*un cas de dépersonnalisation*), thereby abandoning the view that *déjà vu* resulted from a form of 'double consciousness'. Based on a survey undertaken in a 'normal sample' (see Berrios, 1995), Bernard-Leroy (1898) attempted to rekindle the view that a disturbance of recognition was at the core of some forms of the depersonalization, and challenged Dugas' view that it was an independent condition. The latter replied that, because in depersonalization the experience of strangeness encompassed all mental activity (including memories), while in disturbed recognition it was circumscribed, the two phenomena had to be considered as different (Dugas 1898a,b).

Another writer that linked depersonalization to recognition disturbances was G. Heymans (1857–1930), Professor in the history of philosophy, logic, metaphysics and psychology at the University of Gröningen, and first chairman of the Dutch Society for Psychical Research (Sno and Draaisma, 1993). In two student surveys, Heymans found that *déjà vu* was more prevalent than depersonalization, and that the two correlated (Heymans, 1904, 1906). (This has recently been confirmed by Sno and Draaisma, 1993.) The Dutch psychologist saw both as the expression of a common underlying disturbance of *recognition*; and believed that depersonalization was the more severe of the two phenomena. The 'feeling of familiarity', in turn, depended upon the number and strength of associations with earlier memories (Heymans, 1904).

Affect

As early as 1838, Zeller had described patients with experiences of unreality and explained them as resulting from a pathology of affectivity. At a meeting in Berlin, Shäfer reported similar observations: "when these [three] patients complain of their suffering, they relate it explicitly to an emptiness, hollowness in their head, or in the pit of their stomach; of a discomfort of not reaching the surroundings with their inner selves. They, it is true, see and hear everything. But without experiencing any representation (*Vorstellung*) or feeling (*Gefühl*) of their inner stirrings (*inneren Bewegung*), of their sensory vividness (*sinnlichen Wärme*)" (Shäfer, 1880, p. 242). Shäfer considered these cases as a subtype of melancholia, which he called *Melancolia Anaesthetica*.

Störring (1900), in turn, proposed a theory of 'self-awareness' (*Ichbewusstsein*) in which feelings played an important role. Quoting Shäfer, he wrote: [the patients] "have lost the feeling of activity or effort that used to accompany their thoughts and actions, and so they feel in themselves like lifeless machines" (p. 290). Like his French contemporaries, Störring believed that 'coenesthesia' was at the basis of the feeling of 'self-experience': 'organic sensations are a condition of consciousness of self; and the awareness of one's body, which is due to them, must be regarded as one constituent of it'. He also qualified the view by Krishaber and Taine that disturbed perception played a role in the genesis of experiences of self-strangeness. For him, there was a disturbance of the 'power [heightened awareness by the individual] of perception, and accordingly of the awareness that one can have of certain perceptions' (p. 289).

His model included three components (coenesthesia, lack of activity-feelings and power of perception). Combinations thereof gave rise to an altered experience of the self.

On the argument that it captured best the psychological dimension, Löwy replaced Störring's concept of 'activity-feelings' by 'action feelings' (*Aktionsgefühle*). *Aktionsgefühle* was the feeling that accompanied all normal 'psychic activity': "I call it mainly the action-feeling of psychological activity or thought-feeling (*Denkgefühle*), it normally accompanies every psychological act, it provides altogether the awareness of reality of perceived objects … in its absence colours and tones become distant and strange, things become unreal, as from another world" (Löwy, 1908, p. 460). In addition to this general feeling, independent feelings were attached to each psychological function. Thus, there were 'impulse-feelings', when one is aware of an impulse to make a movement, and 'initiative-feelings', when the individual is aware of initiating a choice. Likewise, 'perception-feelings' of bodily and external sensations 'provided the conviction of the existence of our own body'. There were even 'memory feelings' and 'feeling-feelings'. It is important to emphasize that Löwy used the term 'action feelings', to refer to a conscious representation as experience of 'what it feels like to carry out a particular mental activity (including perception), rather than to accompanying emotional feelings like pleasure or dislike'. For example, during the recollection of personal memories, there is, in addition to the information retrieved, a distinct feeling of what it feels like to remember something: a feeling of drawing information from the past. For Löwy, depersonalization was characterized by an absence of 'activity feelings'. The fact that he envisaged the latter as being modality specific, allowed him to explain the clinical observation that depersonalization might be selective in regards to some psychological functions, e.g. patients could complain of being depersonalized in memory, action, perception, etc.

Also, influenced by Störring's concept of 'activity-feelings', Österreich sponsored an 'affective' theory, according to which depersonalization resulted from an inhibition of feelings (*Gefühlshemmungen*): "we postulate that at the foreground [of depersonalization] there is a more or less generalized inhibition of feelings that leads to a reduction of self-feelings and self-awareness"; "this inhibition [also] takes away the feeling of being in control" (Österreich, 1907, p. 37).

Following Janet, Dugas conceived of depersonalization as a failure of conscious integration caused by 'apathy' (Dugas, 1898a,b; Dugas and Moutier, 1911). During the second half of the nineteenth century, this term referred to an abolition of emotions and of psychological energy. This disabled the process of synthesis whereby psychical acts were attributed to the self: "depersonalization … is a form of apathy, if the self is what vibrates and moves, and not what thinks, then apathy is in a sense the loss of the person" (Dugas, 1898b, p. 507).

The fact that Dugas ended up attributing depersonalization to a pathology of emotion may have been influenced by his own overarching views regarding the importance of emotional feelings in the development and expression of personality. Indeed, Dugas strongly believed that emotions were far more important than the intellect in both psychiatry and education. For example, on account of its emotional coldness and exclusive attention to the intellect he called the education of John Stuart Mill 'a complete failure' (Sierra and Berrios, 1996).

Body image

The terms 'body image' and 'body schema' (terms often confused) developed in France and Germany as derivations of the older notions of *cénesthésie* and *Somatopsyche*, respectively (Ey *et al.*, 1947). Body image was meant to make good the fact that *cénesthésie* lacked in 'spatial specificity', the dimension needed to explain distortions of *body* experience such phantom limb or autotopagnosia (Critchley, 1950). Proposed in France by Bonnier (1905), 'body-schema' was taken up by Head to draw attention to the importance of spatial information in the processing of bodily sensations (Head and Holmes, 1911, p. 38). The English neurologists conceived of body schema as a cortical mechanism in terms of which the space-coordinates for the body (as a source of awareness) could be computed.

Schilder's concept of body schema is, on the other hand, embedded in the broader concept of 'body image'. This latter notion is meant to emphasize the experiential aspects of body awareness: 'The image of the human body means the picture of our own body which we form in our mind, that is to say, the way in which the body appears to ourselves' (Schilder, 1935). Merging neuropsychological and psychoanalytical concepts, Schilder suggested that a 'libidinal structure' played a central role in the integration of the body image; and proposed that depersonalization was a disorder of the body image that resulted from defensive re-adjustments of the said 'libidinal structure'.

From a neurological perspective, Ey *et al.* drew attention to similarities between the complaints of depersonalized patients involving parts of their body and those by asomatognosic patients who have lost the representation of a corporal segment. Quoting L'hermitte, they stated (L'hermitte, 1939:) "[the depersonalized subject] sees his body, touches it without being able to persuade himself that it is his own flesh that feels and moves. We are then in the presence of an asomatognosia since the subject sees his body and does not recognise it" (Ey *et al.*, 1947, p. 66). Ey *et al.* shared Schilder's view that emotional factors were crucial to the maintenance of body image, and their pathology played a role in depersonalization: "The image of our bodies is continuously shaped by our sensations and perceptions but emotional processes constitute the energy and force for the constructive synthesis" (Ey *et al.*, 1947, p. 67).

Ehrenwald and Pötzl commented upon cases of subjects with left hemiplegia and anosognosia who went on to develop symptoms resembling depersonalization or Cotard's Syndrome; for example, a patient with a left hemiplegia complained of his left arm as 'being alien (*fremd*), dead, gone away'; he felt a strange hand bigger than the previous one' (Ehrenwald, 1931, p. 683). In three subjects with solutions of continuity in the skull, Hoff and Pötzl (1931) induced feelings of loss of a limb by 'cooling' their right parietal cortex with ethyl-chloride. They were also injected with 'Atophanyl' – believed to have a selective effect upon the thalamus. One of them 'also reported depersonalization – the feeling that it was not him who was talking, as if he was strange to himself, as if talking from another world' (p. 728).

Theories of self-experience

Towards the end of the nineteenth century, the view that 'self experience' was exclusively based on 'sensory information', began to be replaced by the 'active process' hypothesis. Pierre Janet was important in its development. The French psychiatrist wrote: "I have insisted on this essential point. A scientific psychology should consider psychological facts as *actions* and relate to them in those terms" (our italics, Janet, 1928, p. 101). The Janetian model of mind (which originated in Hughlins Jackson) was constituted by a hierarchy of elementary reflexive acts with ever more complex levels of psychological organization. By using this model to explain depersonalization, Janet caused a major conceptual shift in its history.

Janet considered depersonalization as a manifestation of psychasthenia. At the core of this clinical notion, there was the "sentiment d'incomplétude", which referred both to an 'experience of incompleteness' (as reported by some patients with obsessions) and to a broad explanatory mechanism. The complaints of depersonalized patients included reference to 'incompleteness' affecting perception, motor activity, emotions, and feelings of self: "The fundamental feeling conveyed by these expressions is therefore the same as we already dealt with when talking about action, intelligence and emotions, that is, an infinite feeling of incompleteness" (Janet, 1903, p. 318).

The term depersonalization and its related subjective experiences are used by Janet in different ways. The former he uses to refer (in a narrower sense) to 'feelings of incompleteness' as applied to personality; descriptions of the experience (without mentioning the term) he uses to illustrate incompleteness in other psychological domains: "What characterises the feeling of depersonalization, just as the other feelings we have seen, is that the patient perceives himself as an incomplete, unachieved person" (Janet, 1903, p. 318).

In later writings, Janet used the wider term 'feelings of emptiness' to refer to, and explain, *all* the experiences listed in the previous paragraph. By then, his theory of action was fully fledged. He also ascribed the *'sentiment de vide'* to a pathology of action: "The feeling of emptiness is a trouble of action, not of sensation or misunderstood consciousness" (Janet, 1928, p. 101). All psychical activity was either primary or secondary: the former encompassed all activity evoked by external stimuli – from knee jerks to evocation of memories; the latter was a background echo elicited by *representations* of primary acts. By conferring upon primary experiences a 'feeling of vividness' (*l'impression de vie*), this secondary echo created the illusion of a continuous flow of psychic activity: "thousands of resonances, constituted by secondary actions, fill the spirit during the intervals between external stimulations, and give the impression that it is never empty ... This complex activity links up the [primary] actions brutally determined by the external world, and causes an impression of vitality, of spontaneity, and – at the same time – of certitude" (Janet, 1928, p. 126).

Jaspers

Jaspers conceived of the 'self' as a composite of five dimensions: (a) activity of the self, (b) awareness of unity, (c) awareness of identity, (d) awareness of personality, and (e) awareness of self-non-self. A sponsor of the 'self-experience' view, he believed that the 'activity of the self', which mediated the feeling of self-belonging, was crucially affected in depersonalization (Jaspers, 1963, p. 121). Jaspers wrote: "every psychic manifestation, whether perception, bodily sensation, memory, idea, thought or feeling carries *this particular aspect of 'being mine'* of having an 'I' quality, of 'personally belonging', of it being one's own doing. This has been termed *personalisation*" (italics in original; Jaspers, 1963, p. 101). Interestingly, Jaspers' translators rendered this sentence as: 'We have termed this *personalisation*' (Jaspers, 1948 p. 121). (In fact, Jaspers did not use 'we', for he is likely to have been aware that the term had been coined by Dugas in 1911.)

Jaspers then continues: "if these psychic manifestations *(psychischen Elemente)* are accompanied by the awareness that they are not mine, but are alien, automatic, independent, arriving from elsewhere, they are called *depersonalization*" [*so nennt man diese Phänomene Depersonalizationserscheinungen*] (italics in original, Jaspers, 1948, p. 101).

Psychodynamic views

Depersonalization is variously treated by psychoanalytical writers, and it is difficult to offer a unified summary. However, most accounts make use of the hydraulic model of libidinal distribution; for example, Paul Federn (influenced by Brentano, Scheler and Schilder) envisaged the ego as a "homogeneous structure, which is characterized by a specific ego feeling and an ego (self-)experience (Erlebnis)" (Federn 1953; p. 235). According to this psychoanalyst depersonalization and derealization were diseases of the 'ego' caused by a lack of libidinal investment affecting the 'ego structural core' and 'the ego boundaries', respectively. Although Federn conceded that these phenomena might not be clinically specific, he still related depersonalization to schizophrenia, suggesting that they shared (to a different degree) the same psychodynamic mechanism. Indeed, depersonalization might be a premonitory sign of schizophrenia (Federn, 1953). Proposing the opposite, Oberndorf (who during the 1930s wrote about five papers related to depersonalization) believed that an increased libidinal investment in thought processes was central to depersonalization (Oberndorf, 1934). In 1945, summarizing the work of Obendorf, Fenichel explained with his usual clarity: 'the experiences of estrangement and depersonalization are due to a special type of defence, namely to a counter-cathexis against one's own feelings which had been altered and intensified by a preceding increase in narcissism. The results of this increase are perceived as unpleasant by the ego which therefore undertakes defensive measures against them' (Fenichel, 1945; p. 419). Fenichel also quoted Schilder: "persons suffering from depersonalization do not lack feelings; the patients merely perceive, arising from within, an opposition to their experiences" … "an intensified self-observation is the manifest expression of this opposition" (Fenichel, 1945, p. 420).

Indeed, Schilder believed that depersonalization was a developmental syndrome resulting from excessive narcissistic gratification during childhood. Reacting against subsequent deprivation, the subject identified with his own parents and indulged in persistent self-observation during which libido was withdrawn from the outside world: "there is no doubt that in depersonalization the individual loses interest in the outside world and loses with it the interest in his body, which, as has been seen in our previous remarks, has a close relation with the outside world" (Schilder, 1935, p. 140).

Another recurrent psychoanalytical theme has been the view of depersonalization as a defensive process against anxiogenic intrapsychic conflicts (Oberndorf, 1950).

The inter-war period and after

From a more descriptive stance, and according to whether the feelings of unreality and strangeness referred to self or surroundings, Mayer-Gross identified two forms of the condition, and used the term *derealization* to refer to the feeling of alienation of the surroundings (Mayer-Gross, 1935). (Mayer-Gross attributes the term to Mapother but the present writer has been unable to find the published work by the Irish psychiatrist where the term was coined.) Mayer-Gross (already working in Britain at the time) noticed that, in each of these forms of the condition, different mental functions seemed affected, giving rise to a variety of clinical configurations. Although this point had already been observed by Dugas, Löwy, Schilder and others, Mayer-Gross made it with greater force.

The great Heidelberg psychiatrist believed depersonalization to be the expression of a pre-formed functional response of the brain, analogous to delirium, catatonia, seizures, etc.: "It is a characteristic form of reaction of the central organ, which can be set going by different causes. The difficulty of description by means of normal speech, the defiance of comparison, the persistence of the syndrome in the face of complete insight into its paradoxical nature – all these point to something more than purely psychic connections" (p. 118). Because it was seen in the context of most psychiatric, neurological and medical conditions, Mayer-Gross also believed that depersonalization and derealization were non-specific.

Based on his own detailed clinical study of 66 cases of depersonalization, Shorvon contested this view proposing that there was a distinct 'primary' group: "many cases will fit into no other diagnosis than the depersonalization syndrome" (Shorvon, 1946). In a similar vein, Roth proposed the 'phobic-anxiety-depersonalization syndrome' (PADS) defined as a specific anxiety disorder, more common in females, with depersonalization and agoraphobia as its central manifestations (Roth, 1959). Roth also suggested that derealization could discriminate between temporal lobe phenomena and neurotic conditions (Roth and Harper, 1962). However, the fact that PADS eventually came to be understood as equivalent to panic led Roth and Argyle (1988) to reconsider the diagnostic weight of depersonalization within the new category: 'it is plain that depersonalization was given an undeserved prominence in the original description" (p. 39). Following Mayer-Gross, Roth also proposed that depersonalization was a pre-formed brain response shaped by evolution: 'depersonalization comprises a state of heightened arousal together with dissociation of emotion and thus serves as an adaptive mechanism which enhances the chances of survival in acute danger' (Roth and Argyle, 1988, p. 40).

A current classification debate

As can be surmised from the previous pages, perhaps the most recurring theme in the history of depersonalization has been a lack of agreement as to how best to conceptualise and classify the condition. Each proposal has typically emphasized one particular component of the syndrome at the expense of other components. A modern version of the same theme manifests itself in current attempts to classify the condition within current nosological classifications. Whilst depersonalization disorder is classified as a dissociative disorder by DSM-IV, the ICD-10 classifies it as an independent neurotic condition labelled as 'depersonalization-derealization syndrome'. Others in turn have emphasized the anxiety component and see the condition as being closer to an anxiety disorder than to a dissociative one (Hunter et al., 2003). Still others claim that depersonalization is the expression of a qualitatively distinct type of dissociation which differs from that observed in other dissociative conditions (Holmes et al., 2005).

Whether depersonalization is a dissociative disorder or not, is not exclusively an empirical question but very much contingent upon how 'dissociation' is defined. In this regard the conceptual instability of successive DSM definitions of 'dissociation', have at times raised concerns as to the validity of including depersonalization as a dissociative disorder. In DSM-III (American Psychiatric Association, 1980), dissociation was defined as a 'sudden, temporary alteration in the normally integrative functions of consciousness, identity, or motor behaviour'. However, in DSM-III-R, 'motor behaviour' (p. 269) was replaced by 'memory'; but in both versions the inclusion of depersonalization is justified thus: 'Depersonalization disorder has been included in the dissociative disorders because the feeling of one's own reality, an important component of identity, is lost' (American Psychiatric Association, 1987, p. 269). Given the centrality of memory disturbances to the definition of dissociative disorders, the DSM draftsmen felt that they ought to add a cautionary note: "Some, however, question this inclusion because [in depersonalization] disturbance of memory is absent" (p. 269). Such clarification has disappeared from DSM-IV (American Psychiatric Association, 1994) whose definition of dissociation now includes disturbances 'in the perception of the environment' (p. 477) (probably to make conceptual room for 'derealization', as a dissociative disorder not otherwise specified). According to the 'dissociative' view, it was proposed that depersonalization lies on a 'continuum of dissociation' along with other dissociative conditions such as dissociative identity disorder or psychogenic amnesia (Braun, 1984). Other findings, however, do not support a continuum model of dissociation and are consistent with the existence of 'distinct dissociative types' (Putnam *et al.*, 1996). In the same vein, Ross has reported that depersonalization differs from other dissociative states in that it does not occur more frequently in chronic dissociative disorders such as dissociative identity disorder than in panic disorder, and that it is 'the only dissociative disorder that occurs more commonly in partial complex seizures than in controls' (Ross, 1997).

It is clear that both the 'anxiety' and the 'dissociative' view emphasize different valid observations. On the one hand, it is clear that depersonalization disorder has an intimate relationship with anxiety states, which seems specific enough to set it apart from other dissociative conditions. On the other hand, it is clear that the profound disruption of self-awareness which characterizes the condition, can be best conceptualized as being dissociative in nature. In this regard, recent attempts to classify dissociative into two main clinical subtypes is a welcomed and potentially useful conceptual move (Holmes *et al.*, 2005).

(Adapted from Sierra and Berrios, 1997)

REFERENCES

Amiel, H. F. (1933). *Amiel's Journal*, 2nd edn. London: MacMillan and Co.
American Psychiatric Association (1980). *Diagnostic and Statistical Manual of Mental Disorders*. Third edition. Washington, DC: American Psychiatric Associations.

American Psychiatric Association (1987). *Diagnostic and Statistical Manual of Mental Disorders*. Third edition (revised). Washington, DC: American Psychiatric Association.

American Psychiatric Association (1994). *Diagnostic and Statistical Manual of Mental Disorders*. Fourth edition. Washington, DC: American Psychiatric Association.

Bernard-Leroy, E. (1898). Sur l'illusion dite "Dépersonnalisation". *Revue Philosophique de Paris et L'Étranger*, **46**, 157–62.

Berrios, G. E. (1981). Stupor: a conceptual History. *Comprehensive Psychiatry*, **11**, 677–88.

Berrios, G. E. (1996). *The History of Mental Symptoms. Descriptive Psychopathology Since the 19th Century*. Cambridge: Cambridge University Press.

Berrios, G. E. (1995). Déjà-vu in France during the 19th Century. *Comprehensive Psychiatry*, **36**, 123–9.

Billod, M. (1847). Maladies de la Volonté. *Annales Médico-Psychologiques*, **10**, 15–35; 170–202; 317–47.

Braun, B. G. (1984). Towards a theory of multiple personality and other dissociative phenomena. *Psychiatric Clinics of North America*, **7**, 117–193.

Bonnier, P. (1905). L' Aschématie. *Revue Neurologique*, **13**, 605–609.

Critchley, M. (1950). The body image in neurology. *Lancet*, **50**, 335–340.

Critchley, M. (1953). *The Parietal Lobes*. London: Edward Arnold & Co.

Dugas, L. (1894). Observations sur la fausse memoire. *Revue Philosophique de Paris et l' Étranger*, **37**, 34–45.

Dugas, L. (1898a). Dépersonnalisation et fausse memoire. *Revue Philosophique de Paris et l' Étranger*, **46**, 423–425.

Dugas, L. (1898b). Un cas de dépersonnalisation. *Revue Philosophique de Paris et l' Étranger*, **45**, 500–507.

Dugas, L. (1912). Un nouveau cas de dépersonnalisation. *Journal de Psychologie Normale et Pathologique*, **9**, 38–47.

Dugas, L. (1915). La dépersonnalisation, l' illusion du "déjà vu" et celle du "jamais vu". *Revue Philosophique de Paris et l' Étranger*, **79**, 543–555.

Dugas, L. (1936). Dépersonnalisation. *Journal de Psychologie Normal et Pathologique*, **33**, 276–282.

Dugas, L., Moutier, F. (1911). *La Dépersonnalisation*. Paris: Felix Alcan.

Esquirol, J. E. (1838). *Des Maladies Mentales*, Vol. I. Paris: Baillière.

Ehrenwald, H. (1931). Anosognosie und Depersonalisation. Ein Beitrag zur Psychologie der liniksseitig Hemiplegischen. *Der Nervenarzt*, **4**, 681–688.

Ey, H., Ajuriaguerra, J., Hecaen, H. (1947). Troubles de la somatognosie et états de transformation corporelle. In: Hermann, C., editor. *Les rapports de la neurologie et de la psychiatrie (Problèmes neuro-psychiatriques)*. Paris: Actualités Scientifiques et Industrielles, pp. 59–71.

Franck, A. (1875). *Dictionnaire des Sciences Philosophiques*, 2nd edn. Paris: Hachette.

Federn, P. (1953). *Ego Psychology and the Psychoses*. London: Imago Publishing.

Fenichel, O. (1945). *The Psychoanalytic Theory of Neurosis*. London: Kegan Paul, Trench & Trubner.

Foerster, O. (1903). Ein Fall von elementarer allgemeiner Somatopsychose. (Afunktion der Somatopsyche). *Monatsschrift für Psychiatrie und Neurologie*, **14**, 189–205.

Griesinger, W. (1845). *Die Pathologie und Therapie der Psychischen Krankheiten.* Stuttgart: Krabbe.

Griesinger, W. (1868–69). Ueber einige epileptoide Zustände. *Archiv für Psychiatrie und Nervenkrankheiten,* **1**, 320–333.

Head, H. (1911). Holmes G. Sensory disturbances from cerebral lesions. *Brain,* **34**, 102–154.

L' hermitte, J. (1939). *L'image de notre corps,* Paris: Nouvelle Revue Critique.

Heymans, G. (1904). Eine Enquête über Depersonalisation und 'Fausse Reconnaissance'. *Zeitschrift für Psychologie,* **36**, 321–343.

Heymans, G. (1906). Weitere Daten über Depersonalisation und 'Fausse Reconnaissance'. *Zeitschrift für Psychologie,* **43**, 1–17.

Hilgard, E. R. (1980). The trilogy of mind: cognition, affection, and conation. *Journal of the History of the Behavioural Sciences,* **16**, 107–117.

Holmes, E. A., Brown, R. J., Mansell, W. *et al.* (2005). Are there two qualitatively distinct forms of dissociation? A review and some clinical applications. *Clinical Psychology Review,* **25**, 1–23.

Hoff, H., Pötzl, O. (1931). Experimentelle Nachbildung von Anosognosie. *Zeitschrift für die gesamte Neurologie und Psychiatrie,* **137**, 722–734.

Hollander, E., Hwang, M. Y., Mullen, L. S., DeCaria, C., Stein, D. J., Cohen, L. (1993). Clinical and research issues in depersonalization syndrome. *Psychosomatics,* **34**, 193–194.

Hunter, E. C., Phillips, M. L., Chalder, T., Sierra, M., David, A. S. (2003). Depersonalization disorder: a cognitive behavioural conceptualisation. *Behaviour Research and Therapy,* **41**, 1451–1467.

Janet, P. (1903). *Les Obsessions et la Psychasthénie.* Paris: Alcan.

Janet, P. (1928). *De l'Angoisse à l'Extase.* Paris: Alcan.

Jaspers, K. (1948). *Allgemeine Psychopathotologie,* 5th edn. Berlin: Springer.

Jaspers, K. (1963). *General Psychopathology* [Translated by M. Hamilton and J. Hönig from the 5th edition]. Manchester, USA: Manchester University Press.

Kraepelin, E. (1887). Über Erinnerungsfälschungen. *Archiv für Psychiatrie und Nervenkrankheiten,* **18**, 395–436.

Krishaber, M. (1873). *De la Névropathie Cérébro-Cardiaque.* Paris: Masson.

Lamarck, J-B. (1820). *Système Analytique des Connaissances de l'Homme.* Paris: A Belin.

Löwy, M. (1908). Die Aktionsgefühle: Ein Depersonalisationsfall als Beitrag Zur Psychologie des Aktivitatsgefühles und des Persönlichkeitbewusstseins. *Prager Medizinische Wochenschrift,* **33**, 443–461.

Marková, I. S., Berrios, G. E. (2000). Paramnesias and delusions of memory. In Berrios, G. E. and Hodges, J. (eds). *Memory Disorders in Psychiatric Practice.* Cambridge: Cambridge University Press, pp. 313–337.

Mayer-Gross, W. (1935). On depersonalisation. *British Journal of Medical Psychology,* **15**, 103–122.

Oberndorf, C. P. (1934). Depersonalization in relation to erotization of thought. *International Journal of Psychoanalysis,* **15**, 271–295.

Oberndorf, C. P. (1950). The role of anxiety in depersonalisation. *International Journal of Psychoanalysis,* **31**, 1–5.

Österreich, K. (1907). Die Entfremdung der Wahrnehmungswelt und die Deperson-nalisation in der Psychasthenie: ein Beitrag zur Gefühlspsychologie. *Journal für Psychologie und Neurologie*, **9**, 15–53.

Pick, A. (1909). Zur Pathologie des Ich Bewusstseins. *Archiv für Psychiatrie und Nervenkrankheiten*, **38**, 22–23.

Putnam, F. W., Carlson, E. B., Ross, C. A. *et al.* (1996). Patterns of dissociation in clinical and nonclinical samples. *Journal of Nervous and Mental Disease*, **11**, 673–679.

Ribot, T. (1895). *Les Maladies de la Personnalité*, 6th edn. Paris: Felix Alcan.

Ross, C. (1997). *Dissociative Identity Disorder: Diagnosis, Clinical Features, and Treatment of Multiple Personality*. New York: John Wiley & Sons Inc.

Roth, M. (1959). The phobic anxiety-depersonalisation syndrome. *Proceedings of the Royal Society of Medicine*, **52**, 587–595.

Roth, M., Harper, M. (1962). Temporal lobe epilepsy and the phobic anxiety deperson-alisation syndrome. *Comprehensive Psychiatry*, **3**, 215–226.

Roth, M., Argyle, N. (1988). Anxiety panic and phobic disorder: An overview. *Journal of Psychiatric Research*, **22** (suppl 1), 33–54.

Schiller, F. (1984). Coenesthesis. *Bulletin of the History of Medicine*, **58**, 496–515.

Séglas, J. (1895). *Les Maladies mentales et nerveuses*. Paris: Felix Alean.

Shäfer (no initial) (1880). Bemerkungen zur psychiatrischen Formenlehre. *Allgemeine Zeitschrift für Psychiatrie*, **36**, 214–278.

Schilder, P. (1935). *The Image and Appearance of the Human Body*. Kegan Paul, London.

Shorvon, H. J. (1946). The depersonalisation syndrome. *Proceedings of the Royal Society of Medicine*, **39**, 779–792.

Sierra, M., Berrios, G. E. (1996). 'A case of Depersonalization' (by Dugas L., 1898). *History of Psychiatry*, **7**, 451–461.

Sierra, M., Berrios, G. E. (1997). Depersonalization: a conceptual history. *History of Psychiatry*, **8**, 213–229.

Sno, H., Draaisma, D. (1993). An early Duch study of déjà-vu experiences. *Psychological Medicine*, **20**, 22–33.

Sollier, P. (1907). On certain cenesthetic disturbances: with particular reference to cerebral cenesthetic disturbances as primary manifestations of a modification of the personality. *Journal of Abnormal Psychology*, **2**, 1–8.

Sollier, P. (1910). Phénomènes de cénesthésie cérébrale unilatéraux et de dépersonnalisation liés a une affection organique du cerveau. *L'Encéphale*, **2**, 257–271.

Störring, G. (1900). *Vorlesungen über Psychopathologie in ihrer Bedeutung für die normale Psychologie*. Leipzig.

Taine, H. (1906). *De l'intelligence*, 11th edn. Paris: Hachette.

Wernicke, C. (1906). *Grundriss der Psychiatrie in Klinischen Vorlesungen*, 2nd edn. Leipzig: Georg Thieme.

Zeller, A. (1838). Über einige Hauptpunkte in der Erforschung und Heilung der Seelenstörungen. *Zeitschrift für die Beurtheilung und heilung der krankhafte Seelenzustände*, **1**, 515–569.

2

The symptoms of depersonalization

Introduction

The predominant view has been to conceive of depersonalization as a psychological disturbance of self-awareness (Simeon *et al.*, 1997), usually described as a pervasive feeling of unreality. Indeed, although 'feelings of unreality' is still commonly used as a shorthand to describe the phenomenon in clinical practice, its validity as a phenomenological descriptor is more problematic. To start with, it would seem that the term is not used so frequently by patients who are naive to psychiatric discourse (Ackner, 1954; Edwards and Angus 1972). The following observations made by Ackner are still valid:

Unreality is a term which may be employed by patients to describe all varieties of changed experience outside their accepted range of normal variation. Frequently, however, they describe their various feelings of change without at the same time labelling them as feelings of unreality, though they may well agree to do so in direct questioning. Furthermore, one has the impression that the more medical contact the patient has had the more likely he is to formulate his complaint in terms of unreality (Ackner, 1954 p. 846).

Be it as it may, almost all patients struggle to describe the experience, and make use of variety of metaphors which could be classified into two groups. The first kind makes reference to a sense of being cut-off, alienated from themselves and surroundings. For example, patients would often talk about being in a bubble, or being separated from the world by an invisible barrier such as a pane of glass, a fog or a veil (Schmidt, 1951). The second group of metaphors emphasizes instead a qualitative change in their state of consciousness, and complain of feeling as if in 'a dream'…'stoned', 'not awake' or an indescribable 'muzzy feeling', etc. This ineffable aspect of depersonalization sets it apart from other 'neurotic' conditions such as 'hypochondriasis', or 'conversion disorders', where vivid, detailed and often dramatic descriptions are commonplace. It also seems to suggest that, in essence, the condition represents an altered state of consciousness, and as such is indicative of potential neurobiological origin:

What has really been changed or diminished with the onset of depersonalization cannot be expressed in speech. Even educated people (as in some cases in the literature) have given no clearer description, they only used metaphors. Now here is, I think, the point to which the interest of the psychopathologist should be directed. Where normal speech proves unable to deal with an event in consciousness, one may assume that something important is there. Perhaps an underlying brain anomaly makes itself perceptible in this way. Psychopathologists have not bothered very much about this remarkable fact (Mayer-Gross, 1935, p. 106).

Another related regularity in patients' attempts to communicate the experience is the frequent use of 'as if' to qualify their descriptions (e.g. *'I have the feeling as if I am not really here, and as if these were not my hands'* etc.). Such expressions have been traditionally interpreted as evidence of the non-delusional nature of depersonalization. However, the use of 'as if' expressions is more likely to be intended as a critique regarding the adequacy of the description used, rather than as a critique of the reality of the experience itself. Thus, while it is true that patients are painfully aware of the anomalous nature of their experience, they remain convinced that a fundamental, albeit ineffable, change has taken place in them.

Another conceptual problem with the use of 'unreality feelings' as a general descriptor of depersonalization, is that the term introduces a negative definition which has poor explanatory value as it alludes to something missing from normal experience, without clarifying its nature (Sierra and Berrios, 2005; Radovic and Radovic, 2002). As reviewed in Chapter 1, a historical overview of depersonalization clearly shows a pervasive lack of agreement as to the nature of this putative 'missing experience', with different writers pointing to perceptual, emotional, memory or body image related impairments. A common implicit assumption, however, was the notion that the phenomenological complexity of depersonalization could be reduced to the defective functioning of a single mental function.

Depersonalization as a syndrome

An alternative view, that depersonalization could be best conceptualized as a syndrome rather than as a symptom, became well established in the first half of the twentieth century (Sierra and Berrios, 1997; Shorvon, 1946). The following description by Schilder (1928, p. 120), illustrates this:

To the depersonalized individual the world appears strange, peculiar, foreign, dream like. Objects appear at times strangely diminished in size, at times flat. Sounds appear to come from a distance. The tactile characteristics of objects likewise seem strangely altered, but the patients complain not only of the changes in their perceptivity, but their imagery appears to be altered. Patients characterise their imagery as pale, colourless and some complain that they have altogether lost the power of imagination. The emotions likewise undergo marked alteration. Patients complain that that they are capable of experiencing neither pain or pleasure; love and hate have perished with them. They experience a fundamental change in their personality, and the climax is reached with their complaints that they have become strangers to themselves. It is as though they were dead, lifeless, mere automatons. The objective examination of such patients reveals not only an intact sensory apparatus, but also an intact emotional apparatus. All these patients exhibit natural affective reactions in their facial expressions, attitudes, etc.; so that it is impossible to assume that they are incapable of emotional response.

In the above description, Schilder describes four main experiential components, namely: (1) an experience of feeling cut-off or alienated from surroundings (i.e. derealization); (2) difficulties remembering or imagining things; (3) inability to feel emotions, and (4) a feeling of disembodiment, described as a feeling of being dead, or automaton-like. Interestingly, these four symptom domains would seem to correspond broadly with those very mental functions historically deemed relevant to the genesis of depersonalization (see Chapter 1). Another piece of converging evidence comes from a systematic comparison of 200 historical cases of chronic depersonalization, as published in the neuro-psychiatric literature since the late nineteenth century, with 45 current patients with depersonalization disorder. The study revealed the presence of five symptoms, which showed little variation between the historical and modern clinical samples (Sierra and Berrios, 2001): (1) complaints of changes in body experience; (2) automaton-like feelings (i.e. loss of feelings of agency); (3) emotional numbing; (4) changes in the subjective experience of imagery and autobiographical recollections; and (5) complaints of changes in visual perception of surroundings.

In spite of this apparent symptom diversity, it could still be the case that depersonalization results from a single, pervasive experience of detachment equally affecting all aspects of experience. When described separately with regard to emotions, body experiencing, etc., this detachment experience could give rise to the illusion of multiple symptoms. However, the fact that not all symptoms are always present; that some seem more stable than others, or show differential intensity (Sierra and Berrios, 2001) suggests that at least some of these symptoms belong to different experiential domains, with potentially distinct underlying mechanisms (Sierra and Berrios, 1998; Sierra et al., 2002a, b). Furthermore, two recent factor analysis studies using the Cambridge Depersonalization Scale (CDS), support the view that, rather than being a one-dimensional construct, 'depersonalization' represents the expression of several distinct underlying dimensions (Sierra et al., 2005; Simeon et al., 2008). The first study was carried out on 145 depersonalization disorder patients, most of whom had long-standing, constant depersonalization feelings (Sierra et al., 2005). Four well-differentiated factors were found, which were labelled as follows: (1) anomalous body experience; (2) emotional numbing; (3) anomalous subjective recall; and (4) alienation from surroundings (i.e. derealization). Moreover, the fact that an oblique rotation (a statistical factoring model which assumes correlation among factors) yielded a better solution than an orthogonal rotation (a model which assumes independent factors) suggests that the different components of depersonalization represent an integrated response, rather than the mere coexistence of unrelated phenomena. Recently, another research group used the CDS to carry out a confirmatory factor analysis on 450 chronic depersonalization sufferers and obtained a strikingly similar factorial solution (Simeon *et al.*, 2008). They found five factors, four of which clearly overlapped with those found by the earlier study (Sierra *et al.*, 2005). These factors were labelled as follows: (1) 'numbing' (clearly overlapping with the 'emotional numbing' factor of the previous study); (2) 'unreality of self' (which overlapped with the 'anomalies in body experiences'); (3) 'temporal disintegration', a cognitive factor overlapping with our 'anomalies in subjective recall'; and (4) 'unreality of surroundings'. The authors found a fifth factor which they termed 'body distortion'.

To sum up, converging evidence supports the view that depersonalization is a complex phenomenological experience, characterized by the presence of at least four major symptom domains.

The following description from a young patient with depersonalization disorder, known to the author, conveys very well how the different symptoms of depersonalization manifest clinically.

I feel some degree of 'out of it' all of the time, but it has almost become to be what I am used to now. I get times when I feel very out of my body. I am looking at people, know who they are, but can't place myself there. I remember events from the past, but don't always see 'me' there. Even photos of me look different. I don't like the person I remember being. Looking in the mirror proves difficult as I don't always recognize the person looking back at me.

Looking at familiar things during a bad episode upsets me a lot. I look at them, but they just don't seem real, they don't look the same and they don't look familiar any more, even though I know deep down they are, I'm seeing things differently from how I used to, almost like I'm looking at something I know, but it doesn't feel like I know it any more. It feels like I'm looking through someone else's eyes.

I talk and the words are just coming out. I don't feel I have control as to what I'm saying. It's like auto-pilot has been switched on. My voice doesn't sound like 'me' when it is coming out. Sometimes I wonder how I get through conversations as I don't feel I am there at all.

I can sit looking at my foot or my hand and not feel like they are mine. This can happen when I am writing, my hand is just writing, but I'm not telling it to. It almost feels like I have died, but no one has thought to tell me. So, I'm left living in a shell that I don't recognize any more.

I can feel numb of feelings, almost empty inside. I hate the fact I can't feel things as I used to. It's hard with day-to-day life when a lot of the time I struggle to know what is a dream and what real life is and has actually happened.

Anomalous body experience (desomatization)

A substantial proportion of patients with depersonalization disorder describe abnormalities in the way they experience their bodies. Early researchers such as Mayer-Gross (1935) found this symptom to be present in 46% of his series; Shorvon (1946) in turn, reported it in 68% of his 66 patients with chronic depersonalization. A strikingly similar figure (66.2%) was found in a recent series of patients with depersonalization disorder (Sierra and Berrios, 2001). Other early writers, however, believed these feelings to be always present to some degree, although patients might not spontaneously complain about them (Störring, 1933). Differences in the reported frequency of this symptom quite possibly reflect different working definitions and detection thresholds. Unfortunately, most researchers have not provided clear definitions and use vague, generic terms such as 'body alienation' (Mayer-Gross, 1935) or more recently 'desomatisation' (*British Medical Journal*, 1972). In order to describe the different facets of 'anomalous body experience' in depersonalization, it may be useful to subdivide it into several related concepts: (1) lack of body ownership feelings; (2) feelings of loss of agency (the feeling that actions happen automatically without the intervention of a willing self); (3) feelings of disembodiment; and (4) somatosensory distortions.

Lack of body ownership feelings

The experience of having a body is a fundamental aspect of self-consciousness. Such is the need for the 'self' to identify with a body, that a person can be easily tricked into experiencing an externally projected image of a body (Wegner *et al.*, 2004; Lenggenhager *et al.*, 2007), or even a rubber hand of a mannequin (Longo *et al.*, 2008; Tsakiris *et al.*, 2006), as his/her own. For example, a recent experiment involving virtual reality technology was set up in such a way that, when participants wearing goggles tried to look at their own bodies, they saw a mannequin's body instead of their own. Most intriguingly, when they saw the mannequin's abdomen being stroked, while they themselves were stroked in the same region, participants reported feeling as if the mannequin's body was their own (Petkova and Ehrsson, 2008). Patients with depersonalization, in contrast, complain of being unable to experience a relationship between their bodies and the self and experience parts of their body or the totality of it, as alien. A patient with longstanding depersonalization disorder described her experience as follows:

I do not feel I have a body. When I look down I see my legs and body but it feels as if it was not there. When I move I see the movements as I move, but I am not there with the movements. I am walking up the stairs, I see my legs and hear footsteps and feel the muscles but it feels as if I have no body; I am not there. I am sensing that my face and body are not there at all – almost invisible. I see my hands and my body doing things but it does not feel like me and I am not connected to it at all. I don't feel alive in any way whatsoever. I don't feel a thing except for hot or cold; maybe hunger. Even if I touch my face I feel or sense something but my face is not there. As I sense it I have the need to make sure and I rub, touch, and hurt myself to feel something. I touch my neck for instance with my hand but it doesn't feel like my hand touching my neck. I can't feel me touching my own body.... When I move and walk and talk I feel nothing whatsoever. I exercise but don't feel I am doing anything, just my muscles but not my body moving, its madness not to feel myself move, talking...

Interestingly enough, these complaints are reminiscent of those of patients with hemi-asomatognosia resulting from brain lesions. L'hermitte (1939), the famous French neuropsychiatrist, thought this similarity to be so striking that he conceptualized depersonalization as a form of 'total asomatognosia'. Conversely, other authors referred to cases of hemi-asomatognosia as 'hemi-depersonalization' (Ehrenwald, 1931; Critchley, 1953). Typically, patients with asomatognosia have lesions in the parietal lobe and complain about having the sensation *as if* one (usually the left) side of the body did not exist. '*The left arm and leg seem to be "missing" as if the body had been sawn through the vertical midline.*' In less severe cases, the patients do acknowledge the existence of the body part in question, but claim to be unable to experience it as theirs, exactly as do patients with depersonalization. As in depersonalization, patients with asomatognosia ordinarily describe their experience with 'as if' qualifiers (e.g. *as if no left arm and leg existed*). Also, just as is often the case with depersonalization, asomatognosia often assumes the form of a recurring, intermittent phenomenon. Both in depersonalization and in asomatognosia, the patient often has an urge to grope with his good hand so as to palpate the 'missing' limbs as to reassure himself/herself of their existence.

Feelings of 'loss of agency'

Ownership feelings are not circumscribed to the sense of having a body, but pervade all actions. In this context, the term 'feelings of agency' make reference to an experience of owning one's acts and of being an agent of mental and motor activity (Stephens and Graham, 2000). Just as is the case with body ownership, patients with depersonalization frequently complain about an absence of agency feelings so that their behaviour feels automatic, and robotic:

'It's as if a machine was talking to you. Not a person at all, just a mechanical thing or object. I would notice my hands and feet moving, but as if they did not belong to me and were moving automatically'.

It is worth realizing that mental agency seems to be composed of at least two distinct complementary facets: An experiential component, and a cognitive attributional one, by means of which agency is inferred as a by-product of an ongoing self-narrative. For example, as a result of his studies on split brain patients, Gazzaniga has proposed that one of the functions of the left hemisphere is that of creating an ongoing narrative which interprets and generates 'reasonable' accounts for our actions. This putative function has been dubbed as 'the interpreter' (Gazzaniga *et al.*, 1996). It would seem that, in depersonalization, the experiential component of agency is lacking, whilst the cognitive ability to attribute those acts to the 'self' is intact (i.e. agency results from a *post-hoc* reasoning as opposed to direct experience). In contrast, a delusional patient who thinks their actions are being controlled by an external agent seems impaired on both dimensions.

The experience of lacking a sense of agency occupies a central role in the phenomenology of depersonalization (Sierra and Berrios, 1998; Mellor, 1988; Saperstein, 1949). In fact, the very word depersonalization was intended by Dugas to describe incapacity to 'personalize' behaviour (to experience it as belonging to the self) (Dugas and Moutier, 1911, p. 13).

Disembodiment feelings

Disembodiment refers to the experience that the self is localized outside one's physical body boundaries. Unlike the case with full-fledged out-of-body experiences, the typical experience of disembodiment in depersonalization is not usually accompanied by a feeling of occupying a distinct location in extrapersonal space, or by autoscopic hallucinations (Gabbard *et al.*, 1982). Instead, patients typically describe it as a feeling of 'not being there', without any further clarifications pertaining to location in space. In a series of 407 patients with depersonalization disorder 48% were found to endorse an item describing 'disembodiment' on the Cambridge Depersonalization Scale (Sierra and Berrios, 2000): "I have the feeling of being outside my body". More rarely, patients claim to experience themselves in a location outside their bodies and complain that it feels as if their actual self is located at their side, or behind them. Lastly, only a minority of patients (approximately 15%) complain of typical autoscopic experiences, which are characterized by a visual hallucination of oneself as experienced from extrapersonal space. For example, a patient with long-standing depersonalization complained of intermittent out-of-body experiences during which she felt herself to be out of her body, about 1 foot above her head, from where she could see the top of her head. It is likely, however, that such patients suffer from chronic dissociative disorders other than depersonalization disorder.

Somatosensory distortions

This heading encompasses a range of complaints involving actual perceptual distortions of the body. For example, patients complain that body parts, usually their hands, have grown larger or smaller; or that their body feels lighter '*as if walking on a cloud.*' Occasionally, changes in body experience take a more ineffable quality that patients describe by means of metaphors, e.g. '*As if my head was full of cotton wool*'.

Interestingly enough, the above perceptual distortions affecting 'body image' do not seem accompanied by corresponding changes in body schema (defined as unconscious postural and body adjustments regarding motor behaviour) as can be inferred from the following description: "*as I walked I had the distinct feeling of being floating or bouncing up and down on a rubber floor, I wanted to avoid a group of people as I realised they might make fun of my walking. To my surprise they did not seem to have noticed a thing*" (Haug, 1936). Indeed, Cappon *et al.* (1969) marshalled empirical evidence in favour of a dissociation between 'body image' and 'schema'. They compared 20 depersonalized patients and matched controls on different objective tests of body perception, and were unable to find differences between the two groups. It was concluded that "bodily perception may be readily distorted subjectively without affecting the operation of objective judgements or estimates".

Although somatosensory distortions are frequently mentioned in textbook accounts of depersonalization, they do not seem characteristic of depersonalization (Gabbard *et al.*, 1982; Vella, 1965), and may be useful in the differential diagnosis with conditions such as schizophrenia, epilepsy or migraine, where somatosensory distortions are said to be frequent (Priebe and Rohricht, 2001; Rohricht and Priebe, 2002; Watanabe *et al.*, 2003).

Heightened self-observation

A feeling of being a detached observer of one's own behaviour is a noticeable feature of depersonalization, and one that seems intimately associated with the anomalies of body experiencing described above (Schilder, 1935; Sierra *et al.*, 2005). Patients often describe it as a kind of split of their subjective awareness into two minds: one which observes whilst the other goes through the motions: "*...we crossed the street and although my legs moved as I walked, I had the feeling that my mind was elsewhere and from there it observed me... I was unable to know if I was there or if I was the part gone away*" (Roberts, 1960, p. 493).

While some early writers on depersonalization regarded self-observation as an invariable phenomenon and ascribed to it a causal psychodynamic role (Schilder, 1928; Bergler, 1950), other researchers were of the opinion that it only occurred in a minority of patients (Mayer-Gross, 1935; Saperstein, 1949; Shorvon, 1946). Others have made the suggestion that heightened self-observation is secondary to the combined effects of loss of agency and high alertness (Noyes and Kletti, 1977); or that it is the expression of obsessional self-monitoring (Torch, 1981). Given that anomalous body experiences cause the body to be experienced as an object with no relation to self, it is not surprising that heightened self-observation seems correlated with these experiences.

Emotional numbing (de-affectualization)

Most patients with depersonalization report different degrees of attenuated emotional experience, such as loss of affection, pleasure, fear or disgust. Some patients describe an absolute inability to feel and subjectively experience emotions. Other patients, in turn, describe a more subtle impairment characterized by an inability to experience emotional feelings which normally colour perception and mental activity. It has been suggested that such an inability to experience feelings may be causally related to descriptions of things looking 'unreal' (Sierra and Berrios, 1998). Indeed, the narratives of patients often suggest that this might be the case. For example, a patient reported by Brockner (1947) described depersonalization as follows: "*[I am hearing music] but there is no response in me. Music usually moves me, but now it might as well be someone mincing potatoes ... I seem to be walking about in a world I recognise but don't feel. I saw Big Ben alight last night, normally a moving sight to me, but it might have been an alarm clock for all I felt ... My husband and I have always been happy together but now he sits here and might be a complete stranger. I know he is my husband only by his appearance – he might be anybody for all I feel towards him*" (my italics) (p. 969). Such statements would seem to suggest that what is more affected in depersonalization is the ability to imbue perceived objects or concrete situations with emotional feeling, rather than a general inability to experience emotional states (Sierra and Berrios, 1998). In this regard, patients with depersonalization often complain about an inability to experience empathy toward others: "*I just cannot feel anything when somebody else is suffering or in pain. My best friend was diagnosed with cancer a few months ago. We were all telling him how sorry we felt, but I just did not feel a thing, and had to pretend and say all the right words ... It was the same thing when my grandmother died...*". One recent study compared 16 depersonalization disorder patients with 48 healthy controls along a series of tests designed to provide measures of both cognitive and affective empathy (Lawrence *et al.*, 2007). In a short while cognitive empathy reflects the capacity to understand another person's emotional state, 'affective empathy' reflects the ability to experience a congruous emotional response. The main finding of this study was that, while patients with depersonalization showed an intact performance on cognitive empathy, there was evidence of a disruption in the physiological component of affective empathy. Comparable findings emerged from a study looking at the emotional responses to emotive pictures of patients with depersonalization disorder as compared with normal controls and anxiety disorder patients.

Although patients with depersonalization did not experience any difficulties to rate the unpleasantness of pictures on a scale, they showed attenuated autonomic responses to unpleasant pictures and rated them as subjectively less arousing (Sierra et al., 2002a, b).

There are two interesting clinical paradoxes regarding the experience of emotional numbing. The first is that, in spite of their subjective complaints, depersonalized patients show a normal array of emotional motor expressions. In fact, to an external observer they can come across as emotional individuals. Such dissociation is important in the differential diagnosis given that in other conditions in which emotional numbing can be seen, such as in schizophrenia, depression or PTSD, subjective complaints are accompanied by impoverished emotional expression.

The second paradox is the coexistence of complaints of pervasive emotional numbing with those of intense distress and suffering. It goes without saying that a truly, all-embracing, inability to feel emotions, would also preclude the ability to experience suffering. As a matter of fact, however, the very absence of feelings is frequently identified by patients as their major source of distress. Ackner (1954), who like other early writers on depersonalization drew attention to this inconsistency, proposed the idea that the phenomenon could be explained as a consequence of an "increased responsiveness to anxiety of *internal origin*, whereas that of *external origin*, was reduced (my italics, p. 852)." Such differentiation is redolent of a similar one proposed by Sigmund Freud to explain an alleged difference between 'fear' and 'anxiety'. For him, anxiety (Angst) "has a quality of indefiniteness and lack of object. In precise speech we use the word 'fear' (Furcht) rather than 'anxiety' (Angst) if it has found an object" (Freud 1953, p. 165). By object, Freud seems to mean a distinct perception, memory or imagination. This distinction fits in well with clinical observation. Indeed, many depersonalized patients find that, in spite of the significant distress caused by depersonalization itself, previously feared situations or objects before the onset of the condition, fail to elicit any sense of threat or fear.

Anomalies in subjective recall (de-ideation)

Patients with depersonalization disorder often complain of subtle subjective impairments affecting recall and imagery. Although the ability to retrieve information seems unaffected, patients frequently complain that memories, particularly of personal events (i.e. episodic memory) seem to have lost any personal meaning: *"I can remember things, but it seems as if what I remember did not really happen to me"*. Such complaints would seem to correspond to a dissociation between what have been termed the 'know/remember' components of autobiographical memories (Gardiner and Java, 1991). In short, in addition to the retrieval of factual information about a personal event (i.e. a factual or 'know' component), the act of remembering also entails an awareness or particular feeling, that the experience recalled actually happened in the past and is not just being imagined or the memory of a dream. Unlike the case with 'psychogenic amnesias', the 'factual' aspect of the memory is preserved in depersonalization, while it is the 'remembering' component which becomes disrupted, at least in some patients.

Another common clinical observation is that autobiographic memories in depersonalization are usually remembered from a vantage point outside of the body. That is, the event is visualized as if it had been witnessed from outside, rather than through the person's own eyes. This type of memory distortion, which has been called 'observers perspective' remembering (Nigro and Neisser, 1983), has been shown to affect the recall of traumatic situations, or situations which were experienced as threatening (Sierra and Berrios, 1999). Kenny and Bryant (2006) investigated the relationship between memory vantage point and avoidance following trauma in 60 trauma survivors with differing levels of avoidance. It was found that highly avoidant individuals were more likely to remember their trauma from an observer perspective than individuals with a lower level of avoidance. Interestingly, avoidance did not influence the vantage point for positive or neutral memories. These results support the view that the adoption of the observer vantage point for unpleasant memories may serve a distancing, defensive function for people affected by trauma. Similar results have been reported in regards to distressing memories in depression (Williams and Moulds, 2006), and memories related to social interactions in social phobics (D'Argembeau et al., 2006).

Imagery complaints

A related complaint affecting memory is that depersonalized patients often characterize their imagery as pale, colourless or completely absent. Schilder (1914) attributed this phenomenon to an inhibition of visual memory. However, early experimental work showed that recognition of previously seen plates was intact in patients with depersonalization (Störring, 1933). Shorvon (1946) in turn, assessed 16 patients with tests of visual imagery and found that only two seemed to have a genuine and specific impairment of visual imagery. The other patients were found to have non-specific deficits which were ascribed to attentional difficulties. Given the fact that most subjects were found to be 'predominantly visualizers', it was suggested that complaints of lack of imagery were just a way of expressing difficulties to focus attention. One study assessed visual imagery in 28 patients with depersonalization disorder using the vividness of visual imagery questionnaire (VVIQ) (Lambert et al., 2001) and the vividness of movement imagery questionnaire (VMIQ). The former is a 16-item scale consisting of descriptions of visual scenes that the subject is asked to imagine and rate on a 5-point scale ranging from 1= 'perfectly clear and as vivid as normal vision' to 5 = 'no image at all'. The VMIQ in turn is a 24-item scale consisting of movements that the subject is requested to imagine. Using the same 5-point scale as above, the items of this questionnaire request subjects to imagine somebody else performing a movement, and then to repeat the items this time imagining that they are themselves making the movements. As compared with a group of age- and sex-matched normal controls the depersonalization patients were found to have a significant impairment of imagery on both the VVIQ and the VMIQ measures, compared with the controls. Interestingly, patients showed more impairment on the VVIQ with those items requesting to imagine situations involving people as opposed to objects or scenery. On the VMIQ, patients were more impaired at imagining *themselves* making movements, as compared with imagining *another person* making the same movement. In fact, this difficulty to imagine oneself making movements was found to correlate significantly with the intensity of depersonalization as measured by the DES-Taxon ($r = 0.4$ P < 0.01).

A subgroup of ten patients was further tested on a neuropsychological battery of visual perception tests and found to be unimpaired compared with normal controls and patients with obsessive compulsive disorder, despite subjective impairments in imagery (Lambert *et al.*, 2001b).

Complaints of changes in the experiencing of time

Anomalous time experiencing seems commonplace in depersonalization and was well described in the early literature on depersonalization (Lewis, 1931; Schilder, 1936; Oberndorf, 1941). Not surprisingly, however, the reported prevalence of this symptom in patients with depersonalization has been variable. Thus, for some, the symptom was always present (Lewis, 1931; Winnik, 1948; Oberndorf, 1941). For other authors, however, it was only to be found in two-thirds of patients (Shorvon, 1946; Mayer-Gross, 1935). Such differences stem, in all likelihood, from different definitions guiding symptom detection. Most frequently, patients complain that recently experienced events seem to recede into an indefinite remote past. For example, in our series of patients (Baker *et al.*, 2003) 70% endorsed an item of the Cambridge Depersonalization Scale describing this experience: "It seems as if things that I have recently done had taken place a long time ago. For example, anything which I have done this morning feels as if it were done weeks ago."

Other patients complain of more ineffable experiences, such as an inability to experience time, or the experience of existing outside of time. In spite of these dramatic subjective descriptions, it has been found experimentally that the ability of depersonalized patients to provide verbal estimates of time intervals does not differ from normals (Cappon *et al.*, 1969). Lewis (1931) observed a similar dissociation between subjective experiencing and verbal estimations of time. Following Jasper's classification of the psychopathology of time (Jaspers, 1946), it would seem that what is impaired in patients with depersonalization is the 'experience of time' (*Zeiterleben*) as opposed to 'knowledge of time' (*Zeitwissen*). Melges (1982), who wrote extensively on the relation between subjective time and psychopathology, classified anomalous time experiencing into alterations in the sense of duration and of the perspective of time. His contributions to the phenomenology of time experience remain relevant and provide a useful conceptual framework for an analysis of such complaints in depersonalization.

Alterations in the sense of duration

The term '*time sense*' usually refers to the subjective experience of the passage of time (i.e. duration). In this regard, time can be subjectively experienced as going slower or faster than geophysical time (i.e. time as measured by clocks). Researchers have proposed the existence of a putative internal clock as a useful model to account for subjective time experiencing (Cardaci, 2000). Evidence indicates that, if a person's 'internal clock' is going fast, then geophysical time by comparison would seem slow and vice versa (Melges, 1971; Hanke, 2000). In general, hypermetabolic states such as fever, or hyperthyroidism, stimulant and psychedelic drugs, anxiety and manic states are accompanied by an increased speed of the 'internal clock' (Melges, 1982). This in turn, seems determined by an increased rate of mental activity per unit of geophysical time (i.e. the greater the rate of mental activity the longer time duration would seem, and vice versa).

Alterations in the 'perspective of time'

The term 'time perspective' refers to our lineal experience of time as flowing from a future, into a present and receding into the past (Melges, 1982). Anomalies on this dimension of time perception, are typically experienced as if past, present, and future became discontinuous and segregated. For Lewis (1931), distortions in the 'perspective of time' played a central role in depersonalization and he went as far as to ascribe to them a causal role in the genesis of 'feelings of unreality' (Lewis, 1931). In fact, an association between temporal discontinuity and feelings of 'unreality' has been found in a number of studies on patients with both primary and marijuana-induced depersonalization (Melges *et al.*, 1970; Melges *et al.*, 1974; Freeman and Melges, 1977). Of particular interest is the fact that 'anomalies in body experience' were found to correlate with temporal disintegration, hence suggesting an intimate relationship between personal space and time (Freeman and Melges, 1977). Indeed, it might be that the experience of 'time perspective' functions as a frame of self-reference without which the experience of self becomes distorted and unfamiliar (Freeman and Melges, 1978).

The experience of mind emptiness

In addition to complaints of memories seeming pale and devoid of personal relevance; of being unable to evoke visual or auditory images; or of anomalous experiences of time, patients also complain of feelings of mind emptiness, as if they did not have any thoughts (Shorvon, 1946; Schilder, 1914; Sierra and Berrios, 1996). Such experiences are redolent of absorptive states. Interestingly, in the factor analysis mentioned above (Sierra *et al.*, 2005), it was found that the factor 'anomalous subjective recall' correlated significantly with the absorption subscale on the Dissociative Experiences Scale. This relationship would suggest that the experiences subsumed under the term 'anomalous subjective recall' factor may be related to the distorting effect that absorptive states can have on experience and cognition. Patients with depersonalization are often self-absorbed and experience a form of compulsive self-scrutiny, which could affect subjective recall, imagery, and time experiencing (Schilder, 1928; Torch, 1978). Indeed, phenomenological parallels between hypnotic and absorptive states as seen in dissociative disorders, suggest that high hypnotizability (which correlates strongly with absorptive capacity) constitutes a diathesis for pathological dissociative states (Butler *et al.*, 1996). Indeed, recent empirical evidence suggests that hypnotic propensity may be a mediating factor for the experience of depersonalization during panic attacks (Van Dyck and Spinhoven, 1997). In spite of this, a recent study failed to find differences between depersonalization disorder patients and controls on a measure of psychological absorption (Levin *et al.*, 2004). One possible explanation for this is that the instrument used is biased to normative, usually pleasant, involvement in sensory and imaginative experiences. In contrast, heightened absorption in depersonalization is likely to have a negative, self-centred aspect to it, which may have the effect of 'freezing' the mind, rendering attentional and cognitive resources unavailable for creative and open involvement with the world. Also, while the study by Levin *et al.* (2004) looked at depersonalization as a whole, it may be that only a subset of symptoms may be related to increased absorption (Sierra *et al.*, 2005). Simeon *et al.* (2007) recently investigated the relationship between a self-report measure of temporal disintegration and symptoms of dissociation in 52 patients with depersonalization disorder and non-clinical controls. Interestingly, of the three dissociative domains of absorption, amnesia, and depersonalization/derealization, only absorption was a significant predictor of temporal disintegration scores. This would suggest that complaints of temporal disintegration in depersonalization are not directly related to the core symptoms of depersonalization, "but exists when the depersonalized experience involves more prominent absorption" (Simeon *et al.*, 2007).

Patients with depersonalization disorder often complain of attentional difficulties, and the feeling of being overburdened by stimuli. A related complaint is that attention seems to wander aimlessly and would sometimes feel drawn to irrelevant stimuli. Neuropsychological findings do indeed suggest alterations in the ability to 'effortfully control the focus of attention' (Guralnik *et al.*, 2000). Furthermore, intensity of depersonalization has been found to correlate with processing slowness and distractibility (Guralnik *et al.*, 2007). It would also seem that such attentional deficits would have deleterious effects on the short-term memory system. For example, it has been found that patients with depersonalization disorder perform poorly on immediate visual and verbal recall tasks (Guralnik *et al.*, 2007). Thus, in keeping with their subjective complaints, it seems that they have deficits in the ability to take in new information but not in the "ability to conceptualize and manipulate previously encoded information" (Guralnik *et al.*, 2000).

Alienation from surroundings (derealization)

Most patients with depersonalization describe feelings of being cut off from the world around, and of things around seeming 'unreal'. Such an experience is frequently described in terms of visual metaphors (e.g. looking through a camera, mist, veil, etc.). The term derealization was coined in 1935 and ascribed to Mapother by Mayer Gross. After its introduction the usefulness of the concept was soon questioned by experienced psychopathologists on the grounds that its presence was sometimes difficult to ascertain in clinical practice: "[it] does not lend itself to objective distinctions" (Shorvon, 1942). The validity of this observation is still evident in contemporary clinical discussions (Krizek, 1989; Hollander *et al.*, 1990). In fact, it has been suggested that apparent phenomenological differences between depersonalization and derealization might simply reflect different descriptive angles of the same experience rather than different phenomena (Sierra *et al.*, 2005). Dugas, who wrote long before the concept of derealization was proposed, was clearly aware of this descriptive confound: "[in depersonalization] the individual feels a stranger amongst things, or if one prefers, things appear strange to him" (Sierra and Berrios, 1996; p. 456). This notwithstanding, it might be argued that there are genuine phenomenological differences between symptoms pertaining to body, emotional and memory experiencing, and those related to surroundings.

Clinical observations suggest that an inability to experience the hedonic attributes of things perceived is an important feature of derealization (Sierra and Berrios, 1998; Sierra *et al.*, 2005). Indeed, as discussed above, articulate patients frequently ascribe the experience of 'unreality' to an inability to colour experience with pleasurable feelings or feelings of familiarity. Such an observation is supported by the observation that, in the factor analysis described above, an item describing a form of anhedonia loaded on this factor rather than on the emotional numbing factor (Sierra *et al.*, 2005).

'Derealization' commonly accompanies all the other symptom domains of depersonalization disorder, and its isolated occurrence has been questioned or reported as extremely rare. Thus, Coons (1992) reported to have found only two papers which suggested that derealization can occur alone (Rosen, 1955; Krizek, 1989). One study found that, among 44 patients with depersonalization derealization syndrome, only four suffered from 'pure derealization' (Lambert *et al.*, 2000a).

To conclude, this chapter has examined in some detail the phenomenological complexity of depersonalization, and has reviewed converging evidence, which suggests that symptoms of depersonalization can be conceptualized as belonging to distinct, but related psychopathological domains. An understanding of depersonalization in terms of different interacting symptom domains can have important clinical and research implications such as an improved 'caseness' definition and a more precise differential diagnosis with phenomenologically overlapping conditions. From a research perspective, targeting different experiential domains can lead to a better understanding of the condition. It remains to be established if symptom domains can determine clinical subtypes of depersonalization, in just the same way that cases of pure derealization have been reported (Lambert *et al.*, 2001).

REFERENCES

Ackner, B. (1954). Depersonalisation I. Aetiology and phenomenology. *Journal of Mental Science*, **100**, 838–853.

Baker, D., Hunter, E., Lawrence, E. *et al.* (2003). Depersonalisation disorder: clinical features of 204 cases. *British Journal of Psychiatry*, **182**, 428–433.

Bergler, E. (1950). Further studies on depersonalization. *Psychiatric Quarterly*, **24**, 268–277.

Bockner (1949). The depersonalization syndrome: report of a case. *Journal of Mental Science*, **95**, 968–971.

Butler, L. D., Duran, R. E., Jasiukaitis, P., Koopman, C., Spiegel, D. (1996). Hypnotizability and traumatic experience: a diathesis-stress model of dissociative symptomatology. *American Journal of Psychiatry*, **153** (7 Suppl), 42–63.

Cappon, D. (1969). Orientational perception: 3. Orientational percept distortions in depersonalization. *American Journal of Psychiatry*, **125**, 1048–1056.

Cardaci, M. (2000). The mental clock model. Studies on the estimation of time. In Bucceri, R., Di Gesu, V., Saniga, M. (Eds). *Studies on the Structure of Time: From Physics to Psychopathology*. New York: Plenum Pub Corp.

Coons, P. M. (1992). Dissociative disorder not otherwise specified: a clinical investigation of 50 cases with suggestions for typology and treatment. *Dissociation*, **4**, 187–195.

Critchley, M. (1953). *The Parietal Lobes*. London: Edward Arnold.

D'Argembeau, A., Van der Linden, M., d'Acremont, M., Mayers, I. (2006). Phenomenal characteristics of autobiographical memories for social and non-social events in social phobia. *Memory*, **14**, 637–647.

[No author stated] Depersonalization syndromes (1972). *British Medical Journal*, **4**, 378.

Dugas, L., Moutier, F. (1911). *La Dépersonnalisation*, Paris: Felix Alean.

Edwards, J. G., Angus, J. W. (1972). Depersonalization. *British Journal of Psychiatry*, **120**, 242–244.

Ehrenwald, H. (1931). Anosognosie und Depersonalisation. Ein Beitrag zur Psychologie der linksseitig Hemiplegischen. *Der Nervenarzt*, **4**, 681–688.

Freeman, A. M. 3rd, Melges, F. T. (1977). Depersonalization and temporal disintegration in acute mental illness. *American Journal of Psychiatry*, **134**, 679–681.

Freeman, A. M. 3rd, Melges, F. T. (1978). Temporal disorganization, depersonalization, and persecutory ideation in acute mental illness. *American Journal of Psychiatry*, **135**, 123–124.

Freud, S. (1953). 'Inhibitions, symptoms and anxiety', in *The Standard Edition of the Complete Psychological Works of Sigmund Freud*, trans. James Strachey (London: Hogarth Press), **20**, 164–165.

Gabbard, G. O., Twemlow, S. W., Jones, F. C. (1982). Differential diagnosis of altered mind/body perception. *Psychiatry*, **45**, 361–369.

Gardiner, J. M., Java, R. I. (1991). Forgetting in recognition memory with and without recollective experience. *Memory and Cognition*, **19**, 617–623.

Gazzaniga, M. S., Eliassen, J. C., Nisenson, L., Wessinger, C. M., Baynes, K. B. (1996). Collaboration between the hemispheres of a callosotomy patient – Emerging right hemisphere speech and the left brain interpreter. *Brain*, **119**, 1255–1262.

Guralnik, O., Schmeidler, J., Simeon, D. (2000). Feeling unreal: cognitive processes in depersonalization. *American Journal of Psychiatry*, **157**, 103–109.

Guralnik, O., Giesbrecht, T., Knutelska, M., Sirroff, B., Simeon, D. (2007). Cognitive functioning in depersonalization disorder. *Journal of Nervous and Mental Diseases*, **195**, 983–988.

Hanke, W. (2000). Subjective time versus proper (clock) time. In Bucceri, R., Di Gesu, V., Saniga, M. (Eds). *Studies on the Structure of Time: From Physics to Psychopathology*. New York: Plenum Pub Corp.

Haug, K. (1936). *Die Störungen des Persönlichkeitsbewusstseins und verwandte Entfremdungserlebnisse: eine klinische und psychologische Studie*. Stuttgart: Ferdin and Enke Verlag.

Hollander, E., Liebowitz, M., DeCaria, C., Fairbanks, J., Fallon, B., Klein, D. (1990). Treatment of depersonalization with serotonin reuptake blockers. *Journal of Clinical Psychopharmacology*, **10**, 200–203.

Kenny, L. M., Bryant, R. A. (2006). Keeping memories at an arm's length: Vantage point of trauma memories. *Behaviour Research and Therapy*, **45**, 1915–1920.

Krizek, G. O. (1989). Derealization without depersonalization. *American Journal of Psychiatry*, **146**, 1360–1361.

Lambert, M. V., Senior, C., Fewtrell, W. D., Phillips, M. L., David, A. S. (2001a). Primary and secondary depersonalisation disorder: a psychometric study. *Journal of Affective Disorders*, **63**, 249–256.

Lambert, M. V., Senior, C., Phillips, M. L., Sierra, M., Hunter, E., David, A. S. (2001b). Visual imagery and depersonalisation. *Psychopathology*, **34**, 259–264.

Lawrence, E. J., Shaw, P., Baker, D. *et al.* (2007). Empathy and enduring depersonalization: the role of self-related processes. *Social Neuroscience*, **2**, 292–306.

Lenggenhager, B., Tadi, T., Metzinger, T., Blanke, O. (2007). Video ergo sum: manipulating bodily self-consciousness. *Science*, **317**, 1096–1099.

Levin, R., Sirof, B., Simeon, D., Guralnick, O. (2004). Role of fantasy proneness, imaginative involvement, and psychological absorption in depersonalization disorder. *Journal of Nervous and Mental Disease*, **192**, 69–71.

Lewis, A. (1931). The experience of time in mental disorder. *Proceedings of the Royal Society of Medicine*, **25**, 611–620.

Lewis, A. J. (1934). Melancholia: clinical survey of depressive states. *Journal of Mental Science*, **80**, 277–378.

Lhermitte, J. (1939). *L'image de Notre Corps*. Paris: Nouvelle Revue Critique.

Longo, M. R., Schüür, F., Kammers, M. P., Tsakiris, M., Haggard, P. (2008). What is embodiment? A psychometric approach. *Cognition*, **107**, 978–998.

Mayer-Gross, W. (1935). On depersonalisation. *British Journal of Medical Psychology*, **15**, 103–122.

Melges, F. T. (1982). *Time and the Inner Future: A Temporal Approach to Psychiatric Disorders*. New York: Wiley.

Melges, F. T., Tinklenberg, J. R., Hollister, L. E., Gillespie, H. K. (1970). Temporal disintegration and depersonalization during marihuana intoxication. *Archives of General Psychiatry*, **23**, 204–210.

Mellor, C. S. (1988). Depersonalisation and self perception. *British Journal of Psychiatry*, (Suppl.) **2**, 15–19.

Nigro, G., Neisser, U. (1983). Point of view in personal memories. *Cognitive Psychology*, **15**, 467–482.

Noyes, R., Kletti, R. (1977). Depersonalisation in response to life threatening danger. *Comprehensive Psychiatry*, **18**, 375–384.

Oberndorf, C. P. (1941). Time – its relation to reality and purpose: *The Psychoanalytic Review*, **28**, 139–155.

Petkova, V. I., Ehrsson, H. H. (2008). If I were you: Perceptual illusion of body swapping. *PLoS ONE*, **3**(12): e3832. doi:10.1371/journal.pone.0003832.

Priebe, S., Rohricht, F. (2001). Specific body image pathology in acute schizophrenia. *Psychiatry Research*, **101**, 289–301.

Radovic, F., Radovic, S. (2002). Feelings of unreality: a conceptual and phenomenological analysis of the language of depersonalization. *Philosophy, Psychiatry and Psychology*, **9**, 271–283.

Roberts, W. W. (1960). Normal and abnormal depersonalisation. *Journal of Mental Science*, **106**, 478–493.

Rohricht, F., Priebe, S. (2002). Do cenesthesias and body image aberration characterize a subgroup in schizophrenia? *Acta Psychiatrica Scandinavica*, **105**, 276–282.

Rosen, V. H. (1955). The reconstruction of a traumatic childhood event in a case of derealization. *Journal of the American Psychoanalytic Association*, **3**, 211–220.

Saperstein, J. L. (1949). Phenomena of depersonalization. *Journal of Nervous and Mental Disease*, **110**, 236–251.

Schilder, P. (1914). *Selbstbewusstsein und persönlichkeitbewusstsein: eine psychopatho-logische Studie.* Berlin: Verlag von Julius Springer.

Schilder, P. (1928). *'Depersonalization'.* In: *Introduction to Psychoanalytic Psychiatry. Nervous and Mental Disease Monograph Series 50,* New York. Series 50 (pp. 120).

Schilder, P. (1935). *The Image and Appearance of the Human Body.* London: Kegan Paul.

Schmidt, P. (1951). La dépersonnalisation et les limites du moi. *Annales Médico-Psychologiques,* **109,** 408–419.

Shorvon, H. J. (1946). The depersonalization syndrome. *Proceedings of the Royal Society of Medicine,* **39,** 779–792.

Sierra, M., Berrios, G. E. (1996). 'A case of depersonalization' (by Dugas, L., 1898). *History of Psychiatry,* **7,** 451–461.

Sierra, M., Berrios, G. E. (1997). Depersonalization: a conceptual history. *History of Psychiatry,* **8,** 213–229.

Sierra, M., Berrios, G. E. (1998). Depersonalization: neurobiological perspectives. *Biological Psychiatry,* **44,** 898–908.

Sierra, M., Berrios, G. E. (1999). Flashbulb memories and other repetitive images: a psychiatric perspective. *Comprehensive Psychiatry,* **40,** 115–125.

Sierra, M., Berrios, G. E. (2000). The Cambridge Depersonalization Scale: a new instrument for the measurement of depersonalization. *Psychiatry Research,* **93,** 153–164.

Sierra, M., Berrios, G. E. (2001). The phenomenological stability of depersonalization: comparing the old with the new. *Journal of Nervous and Mental Diseases,* **189,** 629–636.

Sierra, M., Senior, C., Dalton, J. *et al.* (2002a). Autonomic response in depersonalization disorder. *Archives of General Psychiatry,* **59,** 833–838.

Sierra, M., Lopera, F., Lambert, M. V. Phillips M. L., David, A. S. (2002b). Separating depersonalisation and derealisation: the relevance of the "lesion method". *Journal of Neurology, Neurosurgery and Psychiatry,* **72,** 530–532.

Sierra, M., Baker, D., Medford, N., David, A. S. (2005). Unpacking the depersonalization syndrome: an exploratory factor analysis on the Cambridge Depersonalization Scale. *Psychological Medicine,* **35,** 1523–1532.

Simeon, D., Gross, S., Guralnik, O., Stein, D. J., Schmeidler, J., Hollander, E. (1997). Feeling unreal: 30 cases of DSM-R-III depersonalization. *American Journal of Psychiatry,* **154,** 1107–1113.

Simeon, D., Hwu, R., Knutelska, M. (2007). Temporal disintegration in depersonalization disorder. *Journal of Trauma and Dissociation,* **8,** 11–24.

Simeon, D., Kozin, D. S., Segal, K., Lerch, B., Dujour, R., Giesbrecht, T. (2008). Deconstructing depersonalization: Further evidence for symptom clusters. *Psychiatry Research,* **157,** 303–306.

Stephens, G. L., Graham, G. (2000). *When Self-Consciousness Breaks: Alien Voices and Inserted Thoughts.* Cambridge: MIT Press.

Störring, E. (1933). Die Depersonalisation: eine psychopathologische Untersuchung. *Archiv für Psychiatrie und Nervenkrankheiten,* **98,** 462–545.

Torch, E. M. (1981). Depersonalization syndrome: an overview. *Psychiatry Quarterly,* **53,** 249–258.

Torch, E. M. (1978). Review of the relationship between obsession and depersonaliza-tion. *Acta Psychiatrica Scandinavica,* **58,** 191–198.

Tsakiris, M., Prabhu, G., Haggard, P. (2006). Having a body versus moving your body: How agency structures body-ownership. *Conscious Cognition*, **15**, 423–432.

Van Dyck, R., Spinhoven, P. (1997). Depersonalization and derealization during panic and hypnosis in low and highly hypnotizable agoraphobics. *International Journal of Clinical and Experimental Hypnosis*, **45**, 41–54.

Vella, G. (1965). Dépersonnalisation somatopsyche et troubles du schéma corporel. *L'Évolution Psychiatrique*, **30**, 147–150.

Watanabe, H., Takahashi, T., Tonoike, T. (2003). Cenesthopathy in adolescence. *Psychiatry and Clinical Neuroscience*, **57**, 23–30.

Wegner, D. M., Sparrow, B., Winerman, L. (2004). Vicarious agency: experiencing control over the movements of others. *Journal of Personality and Social Psychology*, **86**, 838–848.

Williams, A. D., Moulds, M. L. (2006). Cognitive avoidance of intrusive memories: Recall vantage perspective and associations with depression. *Behavioral Research and Therapy*, **45**, 1141–1153.

Winnik, H. (1947–1948). On the structure of the depersonalization neurosis. *British Journal of Medical Psychology*, **21**, 268–277.

3

The depersonalization spectrum

Introduction

Most authors who have written on depersonalization concur on the view that, as a sporadic and fleeting phenomenon, the condition is quite common in both psychiatric and non-clinical populations. For example, in 1964 a panel discussing the clinical relevance of depersonalization concluded that, after depression and anxiety, it was the most frequent symptom seen in psychiatry (Stewart, 1964). Likewise, Paul Schilder (1935), the great German neuropsychiatrist and psychoanalyst, believed depersonalization to be present, at some stage, in 'almost every neurosis', and did not hesitate to refer to the condition as 'one of the nuclear problems of psychology and psychopathology' (Schilder, 1935).

It has long been known that depersonalization occurs along a spectrum of severity, which ranges from short-lasting episodes (so-called 'normal depersonalization') to persistent, severe and disabling forms (abnormal depersonalization). Although depersonalization can frequently accompany other psychiatric conditions (see Chapter 5), in its most chronic and severe form it often follows an independent clinical course. This latter presentation is currently known as 'depersonalization disorder' by DSM-IV or as 'depersonalization-derealization syndrome' by ICD-10. This chapter is intended to provide an overview of these two extremes of the spectrum.

'Normal depersonalization'

A number of studies carried out with college students have clearly established that short-lasting episodes of depersonalization are a common occurrence in young people, with a prevalence ranging from 30% to 70% (Dixon, 1963; Roberts, 1960; Sedman, 1966; Myers and Grant, 1972; Trueman, 1984a,b; Elliot *et al.*, 1984; Moyano and Claudon, 2003). The reported age of onset of these experiences ranged in one study from 4 to 19 with a median of 15 (Roberts, 1960).

Recent surveys on large series of patients with depersonalization disorder have found a similar age of onset (Simeon *et al.*, 2003a). Most studies in non-clinical populations have not found any significant differences in the prevalence of depersonalization between men and women (Sedman, 1966; Myers and Grant, 1972; Roberts, 1960; Dixon, 1963).

Interestingly enough, it has been found that, rather than one-off occurrences, episodes of transient depersonalization tend to be recurrent, which suggests an individual predisposition. For example, in their study on a college population, Sedman *et al.* (1966) found that affected subjects reported a median of five episodes during the previous year, with each episode usually lasting less than 30 minutes. However, in another similar study (Roberts, 1960), subjects reported much longer episodes (mean duration of $5 \pm 3{:}44$ hours). Be it as it may, it was found that the duration of episodes tended to be fairly constant in each individual. It was also established that subjects experiencing frequent depersonalization episodes were significantly younger than those experiencing it as a rare occurrence. Once again, such findings are in keeping with a recent study on patients with depersonalization disorder in which younger age was associated with a more severe course of illness (Baker *et al.*, 2003).

Most cases of 'normal depersonalization' are usually experienced during anxiety-producing situations or low mood. Other commonly accompanying states are characterized by some form of anomalous arousal (65%) such as hypnagogic states; sleep deprivation (Bliss *et al.*, 1959; Cappon, 1968); sensory deprivation (Myers and Grant, 1972; Leonard *et al.*, 1999; Dittrich, 1975; Reed and Segman, 1964; Horowitz, 1964); alcohol withdrawal, and during physical illness and fatigue (Sedman, 1966). Indeed, one study found that the time of onset of depersonalization episodes tended to cluster around evening times (Myers and Grant, 1972). This was interpreted as suggesting a predisposing effect of tiredness. In the same vein, another study found that 58% of participants mentioned fatigue as the most common associated mental state, making it the most common predisposing factor (Roberts, 1960). Subjects frequently stated that they had recently passed through a period of effort, danger, strain or mental concentration. However, rather than experiencing the onset of derpersonalization at the peak of stress, it frequently coincided with the release of tension following the resolution of the stressful situation. Studies focusing on personality factors have found that 'emotional instability' (Myers and Grant, 1972), or anxiety (Trueman, 1984a,b,c) seem to confer vulnerability to depersonalization experiences. In fact, a significant positive correlation was found between the number of depersonalization episodes and scores on an anxiety scale (Trueman, 1984a,b,c).

Phenomenology

A phenomenological analysis of transient depersonalization experiences as reported in student samples, seems to suggest that, with the exception of

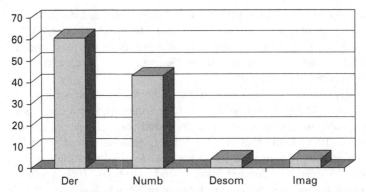

Fig. 3.1. Symptom profile of depersonalization experiences as reported by college students experiencing transient depersonalization episodes (Myers and Grant, 1972). Numbers are percentages of patients reporting each symptom domain.

Abr: Der = Derealization; Numb = Emotional Numbing; Desom = Desomatization; Imag = Subjective deficits in visual imagery.

derealization and emotional numbing, the reported frequencies of other symptom domains are substantially lower than those found in subjects with pathological depersonalization (Myers and Grant, 1972). Such a finding is interesting, in that it has been found that, whilst derealization is present even in mild cases of depersonalization disorder, the other components of the syndrome, in particular 'anomalies in subjective experience' show a more linear relationship with overall depersonalization severity. In other words, it would seem that the symptom profile of 'normal depersonalization' resembles that of mild intensity depersonalization disorder patients. Thus, it would seem that the difference between 'normal' and 'pathological' depersonalization lies not only in the sporadic and fleeting nature of episodes in the former, but also in less severe symptom intensity.

Depersonalization in the general population

A recent epidemiological study in a southern rural US sample of 1008 households representative of the general population found a 1-year prevalence for depersonalization and derealization to be 19.1% and 23.4%, respectively (Aderibigbe et al., 2001). The prevalence for either phenomenon was 23.4%. In keeping with the college-based studies discussed above, it was found that the highest prevalence of depersonalization/derealization (38.1%) occurred in the age group 18–22, and progressively declined in older groups. In general, the prevalence of depersonalization/derealization was significantly higher in females (26.5 vs. 19.5 in men).

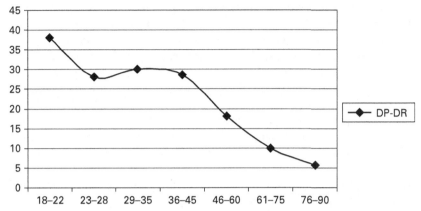

Fig. 3.2. Prevalence distribution of depersonalization-derealization experiences in different age groups (data taken from Aderibigbe *et al.*, 2001).

It was found that 80% of those reporting depersonalization/derealization experiences (19% of the total general population), admitted to more than three episodes in the previous year, or had episodes lasting more than 1 hour. Thus, in keeping with studies in college populations, these findings suggest that, in those predisposed, depersonalization rarely happens as a one-off experience.

Interestingly, those respondents suffering from chronic pain were found to be almost three times more likely to experience depersonalization/derealization than those who did not. An association between clinically significant depersonalization and chronic pain has also been found in an epidemiological study on the German population (Michal *et al.*, 2009).

Other apparent precipitants seemed specific for either depersonalization or derealization. For example, while depersonalization was found to be weakly associated with severe stress, anxiety or low mood, derealization did not seem to have any obvious triggers with the exception of perceived danger (Aderibigbe *et al.*, 2001).

'Pathological depersonalization'

As discussed above, it would seem as if the spectrum of intensity that seems to characterize depersonalization occurs along at least four dimensions of severity: frequency and duration of episodes, subjective intensity and number of symptoms involved. Thus, as one moves from one extreme of the continuum to the other, episodes become more frequent, longer lasting, and seem to encompass more symptom domains. It has also been suggested that depersonalization precipitants vary along the continuum. According to Steinberg (1995), 'common-mild depersonalization', defined as 'one or few episodes', lasting 'seconds to minutes', typically would be triggered by extreme fatigue, sensory deprivation, medical illness, drug or alcohol intoxication, sleep deprivation and severe psychosocial stress. However, these triggers would not seem as relevant when it comes to pathological depersonalization and, although it can be precipitated by stressful events, the condition can become chronic even in the absence of identifiable stress (Steinberg, 1995). It is likely, however, that in many cases pathological depersonalization is usually a comorbid manifestation of other distressing concomitant conditions, either mental or physical (Steinberg *et al.*, 1991). In a large epidemiological study on the general population, researchers found a high association between 'clinically significant depersonalization' and both anxiety disorders (68%) and depression (52%) (Michal *et al.*, 2009). Such findings are very much in keeping with the high prevalence of depersonalization among psychiatric patients (Hunter *et al.*, 2004). For example, Brauer *et al.* (1970) studied the prevalence of depersonalization in 212 psychiatric in-patients, and found that 80% admitted to present or past depersonalization experiences. However, only 12% reported severe and lasting experiences. A similar high prevalence has been found recently in a transcultural study of depersonalization among psychiatric in-patients (Sierra *et al.*, 2006). A strong, independent association has also been found recently between pathological depersonalization and self-reported somatic diseases such as hypertension, diabetes mellitus, chronic pulmonary disease and chronic pain (Michal *et al.*, 2009). This association seemed specific and not accounted for by associated depression or anxiety. Interestingly, the authors found that, as compared with participants with a mental disorder but without depersonalization, those reporting depersonalization reported lower subjective health, greater work incapacity, and higher use of psychotherapy and psychotropic medications (Michal *et al.*, 2009). Such findings are in keeping with findings suggesting that depersonalization is associated with higher morbidity and disease severity of comorbid conditions (Mula *et al.*, 2008).

'Depersonalization disorder'

Pathological depersonalization which seems 'independent' from comorbid conditions is currently labelled by DSM-IV as 'depersonalization disorder' (APA, 1994) and by ICD-10 as 'depersonalization-derealization syndrome' (WHO, 1992). This concept of nosological independence does not preclude the existence of comorbid conditions, but requires that depersonalization 'not only occurs in their presence'. For example, although a patient may have suffered from panic disorder at some stage, if depersonalization occurs at times when the patient is not suffering from anxiety attacks, then a diagnosis of depersonalization disorder is legitimate. Such a pragmatic approach certainly bypasses the clinical conundrums of trying to establish whether depersonalization is primary or secondary to a concomitant or pre-existing condition.

As reviewed in Chapter 1, Shorvon (1946) was the first to propose that chronic depersonalization constituted a psychiatric illness in its own right. He published a series of 66 patients affected by chronic depersonalization, in whom no other underlying diagnosis could be identified. The following case illustrates well the main clinical features of the condition.

The patient is a 27-year-old male, who claimed to have been well until the age of 20, when his symptoms began: "One day as I was on the train, I suddenly started feeling very weird and different, as if I was dreaming and not really there." This ineffable mental state continued with little variation and in fact remained unabated for the following 7 years. He described his symptoms as a constant feeling of unreality, and also complained of an inability to experience emotions subjectively. He claimed that his body felt very alien to him, and he had a constant feeling of being on automatic pilot. Additionally, he complained of having lost the ability to experience hunger or thirst, and noticed that other visceral feelings such as wanting to urinate were not consciously experienced as before, and only registered as a vague sense of discomfort. It was similar with his ability to feel pain in that he failed to experience any associated emotional suffering: "I can feel the pain, but it is as if I don't care, as if it was somebody else's pain". He also claimed to have lost the ability to feel physical tiredness. Other related symptoms were a severe inability to visualize things with his mind's eye and an altered sense of the passage of time. He found the latter most difficult to describe: "it feels as if time does not mean anything; as if I exist outside time." He also stated that personal memories felt unrelated to him "I remember things but it does not feel as if I was there".

He thought that his symptoms started at a time when he was feeling rather 'stressed out' in his second year at university. Shortly after the onset of depersonalization, he had to give up his university studies, as he felt depersonalization made it impossible for him to perform to required standards.

There was no family history of mental illness. He claimed to have had happy memories from childhood, although he had been sent to a boarding school since a very early age. There was no history of physical or sexual abuse.

Mental status examination did not reveal any comorbid psychiatric condition. Neurological examination, screening blood tests, as well as a brain MRI and EEG proved unremarkable.

He had been previously tried on a number of new generation antidepressants as well as olanzapine, but he did not experience any benefits.

Administered scales yielded the following:

Cambridge Depersonalization Scale: 162 (in the range of severe depersonalization)
Dissociative Experiences Scale: 18 (within normal range)
Beck's Anxiety Inventory: 12 (within normal range)
Beck's Depression Inventory: 21 (in the range of mild depression).

This patient was found clearly to meet criteria for a diagnosis of DSM-IV depersonalization disorder or ICD-10 Depersonalization-Derealization Syndrome. Although he scored in the range of moderate depression on the Beck's Depression Inventory, the endorsement of items was more a reflection of subjective distress than of a concomitant depressive syndrome.

In the last decade, two independent, large series of patients meeting criteria for depersonalization disorder have been studied in the US and the UK. The findings, as it pertains to demographics, onset, course of illness and clinical profile are strikingly similar and very much in agreement with previous series. The following section offers a summary of those findings.

Demographic profile

It has been found that the condition is equally distributed between genders. Affected individuals at the time of diagnosis tend to be in their 20s or 30s but the onset of the condition is usually reported as dating back to the late teens or early 20s (Baker *et al.*, 2003; Simeon *et al.*, 2003a). In one series of 204 patients, 62% were found to be single at the time of diagnosis, and 38% were unemployed. Another study on a large series of patients found a similar demographic profile (Simeon *et al.*, 2003a). Most patients complain that the condition prevents them from taking up employment, or performing at a level commensurate with their training or intellectual abilities. Similarly, most feel that the condition makes it difficult to commit to a long term relationship (Simeon, 2004).

Onset of depersonalization disorder

The onset of depersonalization disorder is usually during adolescence or early adulthood, with the majority of cases claiming that the condition began between the ages of 15 and 19 (Baker *et al.*, 2003; Simeon *et al.*, 2003a). In fact, 30% of patients report an onset before the age of 16, and 5.6% claim that depersonalization started between the ages of 4 and 10 (Baker *et al.*, 2003). Although such cases are subject to criticism on the grounds of possible memory distortion or false memories (Toglia *et al.*, 1999), genuine cases of childhood depersonalization have been reported (Salfield, 1958, 1957; Eggers, 1979). In fact, it has been suggested that the apparent paucity of depersonalization cases during childhood reflects an underreporting effect. Lack of detection could be a result of the reduced linguistic abilities of children, which would make it almost impossible for them to describe the experience (Meyer, 1961; Salfield, 1958). In this regard, it has been found that, whilst adults often resort to metaphors to describe the experience, children tend to use similes (Shimizu and Sakamoto, 1986).

An adult patient seen by the author claimed that her condition started suddenly at the age of 7: "*I remember exactly the day when it happened; I had been swimming that day and then, suddenly, I started feeling extremely odd. In retrospect I can see it was the same feeling I have now. I felt so strange, but did not have the words to describe it. I was distressed and when my mother asked me what was wrong, all I could say was that my swimming suit did not seem to fit.*" More than 20 years later, she still struggles to convey her ongoing experience: "*I find it difficult to describe my symptoms. I feel detached and isolated from the world and the people in it. I feel like I am in a box of very thick glass which stops me from feeling any atmosphere. At times it is like looking at a picture. It has no real depth. I'm like a zombie unable to take in any information.*"

Another patient claiming to remember episodes of depersonalization when he was 7 described them as follows: "*I would call my mum describing that I was 'having a feeling'. This feeling was inexplicable and the only way I could describe it at the time was that a dark sensation would spread over me and I would have no idea who I was or where I was, I could find no familiarity in anything.*"

The finding that, in most cases, depersonalization disorder seems to begin during childhood or adolescence finds further confirmation from the fact that its onset after middle age is extremely rare. One study found that only 5% of 117 patients reported an onset of the condition after the age of 25 and there were no cases with onset after 40 (Simeon *et al.*, 2003a). Similarly, another study found that 28.4% of 204 cases experienced onset after 25 years of age, and only 8% after 40 (Baker *et al.*, 2003). Interestingly, it was found that an early-onset group (0–16) had significantly higher depersonalization scores than a mid-onset group (17–39), which, in turn, scored higher than a late-onset group (>40). It is clear that any theory attempting to explain the nature of the depersonalization should be able to account for the striking consistency of onset around the time of puberty and adolescence. It has been suggested that identity restructuring during adolescence may predispose to depersonalization experiences (Meares and Grose, 1978). More specifically, one study looked into the relationship of self-esteem and self-awareness with depersonalization in a sample of 352 adolescents aged 12–16 (Roth, 1998). It was found that those predisposed to episodes of depersonalization were more self-conscious than their non-affected counterparts. This is an interesting observation in light of recent studies showing a strong relationship between depersonalization disorder and social anxiety (Michal *et al.*, 2005b).

In approximately half of all cases depersonalization disorder begins suddenly, and patients often describe the experience 'as if somebody had flicked a switch' in their heads. In such cases patients give vivid accounts of the event and the circumstances surrounding it, such as thoughts or conversations they were having at the time, time of the day, etc.

"*I remember I was at the university library reading a book. All of a sudden I felt as if something threatening and deathly brushed past me… it felt like the flick of a switch. Everything in the library remained the same, but I felt utterly changed from that moment on …*"

"*It happened one evening in the late summer of 1998 as I was playing tennis with a friend. Quite suddenly, I experienced a sense of looking around me and feeling that everything seemed unreal...I didn't feel dreamy but as if I was physically not quite there. It was as if I was looking through a pane of glass or out of a television screen."*

In other patients the onset seems more gradual and they are unable to state with any certainty when it was that the condition began. Be it as it may, the onset of depersonalization is usually experienced with great distress, and most patients harbour fears of going mad, or of having a serious neurological condition (Hunter *et al.*, 2005).

In many cases the onset of depersonalization disorder coincides with a period of emotional upheaval and stress. Frequently, patients feel trapped by circumstances, and as if they have lost all control. In fact, it would seem that perceived threat and external locus of control are a common denominator to most triggers. Interestingly, it is not uncommon to observe that the onset of depersonalization brings about an attenuation of concomitant anxiety. For example, a patient whose depersonalization onset had been preceded by a mounting constant anxiety during the previous year, woke up one morning experiencing full blown depersonalization. *"I felt disoriented, as if I was in a dream, I did not feel me anymore. It felt as if I had been taken to another planet where everything looked strange and unfamiliar."* Although she found this state extremely distressing, she found that, in a strange and paradoxical way, she could no longer experience anxiety as she had before the onset of the condition. In those cases in which the onset of depersonalization coincides with a period of frequent panic attacks, the emergence of constant depersonalization is often accompanied by a significant reduction of panic attacks. This 'filtering-out' effect of depersonalization has been observed in regards to other preceding symptoms, including physical fatigue, obsessions and low mood.

Course of illness

Depersonalization disorder is a chronic condition. In one large series the mean duration was found to be around 14 years (Baker *et al.*, 2003). In about two-thirds of patients, depersonalization is constant, although it may fluctuate in intensity. Usually stressful situations, fatigue, sleep deprivation and alcohol hangover make it worse, while relaxing situations or cognitive distraction make it more tolerable. Some patients relate the rare occurrence of sudden 'symptom-free' gaps, which unfortunately last only a few seconds in most cases.

In one-third of patients depersonalization disorder runs an episodic course, with each episode usually lasting from a few days to a few months (Simeon *et al.*, 2003a; Baker *et al.*, 2003). In a significant proportion of patients, depersonalization starts episodically, and may continue so for weeks or months before becoming constant (Baker *et al.*, 2003; Simeon *et al.*, 2003a).

Psychiatric comorbidity of depersonalization disorder

Patients frequently complain of significant anxiety symptoms and low mood. In a systematic assessment of comorbid conditions, it was found that, among their 117 patients with depersonalization disorder (Simeon *et al.*, 2003a), the 'current' prevalence of affective and anxiety disorders was as follows: bipolar mood disorder = 1.7%; major depression = 10.3%; panic disorder = 12%; social phobia = 28.2%. None of these disorders was found to have pre-existed before the onset of depersonalization (Simeon *et al.*, 2003a).

Moreover, the presence of comorbid conditions was not found to predict the severity of depersonalization symptoms. The same authors found that approximately 60% of their patients had a comorbid personality disorder (Simeon *et al.*, 2003a). Although all personality disorders were represented in the series, the most frequent were 'borderline' (21%); 'avoidant' (23%) and 'obsessive-compulsive' (21%). In general, the above findings support the view that depersonalization disorder represents a condition in its own right, and is not just the manifestation of atypical anxiety or mood disorders (Simeon, 2004).

The prevalence of depersonalization disorder

A number of recent studies using validated instruments suggest that the prevalence of depersonalization disorder in the general population may not be unlike that of schizophrenia or manic depressive illnesss. In one study, researchers administered the Dissociative Disorders Interview Schedule to a representative sample of the population in Canada and found that the prevalence of abnormal depersonalization was 2.5% (Ross *et al.*, 1990).

Another group of researches recently carried out a 'representative face-to-face household survey' on a sample representative of the general German population (*n* = 1287) (Michal *et al.*, 2009). The main finding of this study was that 1.9% obtained scores within the range of clinically significant depersonalization on an abridged version of the Cambridge Depersonalization Scale. Their findings allowed the authors to conclude that "depersonalization is common, it can not be reduced to a negligible variant of depression or anxiety and that more awareness about depersonalization with respect to detection and research is urgently required" (Michal *et al.*, 2009).

In yet another study, a representative sample of 658 individuals from New York state were assessed by means of a semi-structured clinical interview derived from the items in the DES-T and selected SCID-D items (Johnson *et al.*, 2006). The 1-year prevalence for depersonalization disorder was 0.8%. In spite of the above findings, the belief that depersonalization disorder is an extremely rare condition is still rife amongst psychiatrists. In fact, such an assumption is currently enshrined in the ICD-10, which defines 'depersonalization-derealization syndrome' as '*a rare disorder*'. Even more striking is the fact that depersonalization disorder is currently listed as a 'rare disease' by the Office of Rare Diseases (ORD, 2007) of the National Institutes of Health (NIH). Their definition of 'rare disease' is currently operationalized as any condition affecting less than 200 000 people in the US population, a prevalence far lower than those revealed by the epidemiological studies mentioned above.

The reasons for the discrepancy between research findings and clinical experience may be severalfold:

(1) Psychiatrists are still trained to believe that depersonalization disorder is extremely rare or non-existent and that, when present, it is usually a secondary, almost irrelevant symptom of another condition such as depression or anxiety. Not surprisingly, this received view leads to a high rate of misdiagnosis. The types of erroneous diagnoses are usually depression, anxiety disorders, atypical psychosis, and temporal lobe epilepsy (Baker et al., 2003; Simeon et al., 2003a). Studies have shown that the average time from onset of the condition until it is diagnosed is of 7–12 years (Hunter et al., 2003).

(2) Another possible reason for the belief that depersonalization disorder is rare is that many patients may not look for help. In fact, it is not unusual for patients to keep their symptoms secret from friends and family. Such reluctance to talk stems from the ineffable nature of the condition and the accompanying difficulty patients experience describing it (Edwards and Angus, 1972); and from fears of being thought 'mad' by others (Simeon, 2004).

(3) Another possible explanation for the discrepancy between clinical experience and epidemiological findings could be found in what has been termed in epidemiological literature as the 'clinician's illusion'. The latter constitutes a bias arising from the fact that those patients seen by clinicians constitute a particular subgroup, whose members differ in important respects to those found in community-based samples (Cohen and Cohen, 1984). One way in which the two groups may vary is in the amount of distress or impairment which accompanies depersonalization. For example, one study analysed in detail a non-clinical sample of 20 individuals suffering from depersonalization 'either in a continuous or sporadic form', none of whom suffered from any other comorbid condition (Charbonneau and O'Connor, 1999). Although both the age of onset (20.8 ± 12.4) and the duration of depersonalization (16.9 ± 13.7 years) were very similar to those reported in clinical samples of depersonalization disorder (Baker et al., 2003; Simeon et al., 2003a), only three participants admitted to significant enough subjective distress to justify a DSM-IV diagnosis of depersonalization disorder. In fact, 3 out of the 20 participants even claimed to find depersonalization an enjoyable experience. Likewise, in their epidemiological survey on the German general population, researchers found that 4 of their 25 subjects with clinically significant depersonalization did not admit to any accompanying distress (Michal et al., 2009).

Predisposing factors

Recent studies have shown that patients with depersonalization disorder report significantly more traumatic experiences than healthy controls (Simeon *et al.*, 2001b). In particular, a history of 'emotional abuse' in childhood (p. 121) was found to predict depersonalization severity. A similar association between depersonalization and emotional abuse has been recently documented in a sample of normal controls and patients attending a psychosomatic specialized clinic on account of chronic pain (Michal *et al.*, 2007). It has also been found that, in patients with panic disorder, those who depersonalize during panic attacks report more history of trauma as compared with those who do not depersonalize (see Chapter 5). Similarly, it has been found that patients with borderline personality disorder prone to dissociative experiences also report more experiences of 'emotional abuse' compared with those who don't dissociate (Simeon *et al.*, 2003b). In fact, it would seem that a history of 'emotional abuse' constitutes a risk factor for the development of personality disorders, a relevant finding given the extensive comorbidity between depersonalization disorder and personality disorders. It would seem that patients with depersonalization disorder exhibit a personality structure characterized by immature psychological defences, and by a significantly higher 'harm-avoidant' temperament, as compared with healthy controls (Simeon *et al.*, 2002). It was further found that those defensive traits correlated with the intensity of dissociative experiences.

The diagnosis of depersonalization

Although depersonalization is often described in terms of 'feelings of unreality', it can be misleading to rely on this term for diagnostic purposes as discussed in the previous chapter.

A more universal finding in patients with depersonalization is the ineffable quality of the experience and the corresponding difficulty to articulate it in words. As discussed in Chapter 2, most patients use metaphors or similes which emphasize either a sense of 'separation', and being cut-off, or that of being in an altered state of consciousness such as being 'in a dream', 'as if I am not really awake', etc.

In view of the entirely subjective nature of depersonalization, the difficulties experienced by patients to describe it, and their reluctance to talk about 'bizarre' sounding experiences, it is important to devote time and effort to explore its phenomenology in detail as part of the diagnostic process.

Edwards and Angus (1972) aptly commented that the diagnosis of depersonalization *"is not just a reflection of the skill of the interviewer, but is dependent on the type of questions and the manner in which they are asked. The less structured the interview, the more likely it is that there will be inconsistencies in the frequency with which depersonalization is recognized"* (p. 243).

In view of the syndrome-like structure of depersonalization, it seems a good idea to structure the interview along the four symptom domains discussed in the second chapter. Patients are often hesitant and guarded when it comes to describing their symptoms, and often make pre-emptive statements such as "you are probably going to think I am mad but…" or would interrupt a description with a question such as "does this make any sense to you?" In this respect, it can be useful to make an indirect emphatic acknowledgement of the ineffable aspect of depersonalization by asking the patient something along the lines of: "How difficult is it to describe what you are experiencing now?; How would you describe it?" Given the metaphor abundance of most replies, it may at times be difficult to decide, as Ackner (1954) stated, how much "objective reality there is in the word or how much metaphor", or how the latter is to be understood. In such instances it is useful to ask directly for clarification rather than taking the description at face value. For example: "Is that actually the way you experience this, or just a way in which you try to communicate it?" Such slight challenges to offered descriptions are often useful in unveiling new information. In my experience, chronic depersonalization sufferers usually present their symptoms by means of highly rehearsed description, often plagued with technical or 'textbook' terms. This is not surprising, given the currently available access to relevant websites and discussion forums. One long-standing depersonalization disorder sufferer acknowledged this: "it has taken me years to learn how to describe what I feel". It is then useful to ask for clarifications, daily life examples, and alternative ways of describing the experience.

Depending on which symptom domains are spontaneously emphasized by the patient, probing questions should proceed to explore omitted symptom areas. For example, to a patient spontaneously describing 'derealization', one could ask: "Has this affected your emotions or your ability to feel in any way? What about the way you experience your body?; Are there any changes in the way you experience memories of things which have happened to you?"

Another useful way to explore depersonalization symptoms is to administer a phenomenologically comprehensive scale such as the Cambridge Depersonalization Scale (more on this scale below), and then, focusing on those items which the patient has endorsed, to ask for daily life examples in which the experience in question has occurred.

Rating scales and structured interviews

A number of self-rating scales have been developed for the purpose of assessing depersonalization. Although some of them have proved able to discriminate between patients with depersonalization disorder and healthy controls (Simeon *et al.*, 1998), they either show dubious face validity or fail to address the phenomenological complexity of depersonalization (Sierra and Berrios, 2000). Other relevant, promising scales are still in need of further validation research (Cox and Swinson, 2002; Simeon *et al.*, 2001a).

Based on a comprehensive study of the phenomenology of depersonalization Sierra and Berrios (2001) developed a self-rating scale which was shown to differentiate patients with depersonalization disorder from patients with temporal lobe epilepsy and with anxiety disorders.

Cambridge Depersonalization Scale (see Appendix)

The Cambridge Depersonalization Scale (Sierra and Berrios, 2000) is a comprehensive instrument containing 29 items describing experiences classically associated with the depersonalization syndrome. It is the most comprehensive scale on the phenomenology of depersonalization and has been used increasingly in depersonalization-related research. It shows a good to excellent psychometric profile (see below) and its use in treatment trials has shown it to be sensitive to change (Hunter *et al.*, 2005; Sierra *et al.*, 2006; Simeon *et al.*, 2005). Its items have been shown to segregate along four distinct dimensions classically associated with depersonalization: (1) anomalous body experiences; (2) emotional numbing; (3) anomalies in subjective recall; (4) derealization (Sierra *et al.*, 2005). A confirmatory factor analysis revealed a very similar factorial solution, but added a fifth factor of 'body distortion' (Simeon *et al.*, 2008).

Each item of the CDS is rated on two Likert scales for frequency and duration of the experience. Given that depersonalization symptoms can be intermittent, the scale was designed so that the arithmetic sum of frequency and duration yields an index of item intensity (range 0–10). In this way, the clinically valid observation is saved that a patient experiencing frequent but short lived depersonalization experiences should be rated as suffering from an equivalent degree of intensity to someone having less frequent but long-lasting experiences. The global score of the scale is the arithmetic sum of all items (range 0–290). The CDS was initially validated on patients with depersonalization disorder, and was shown to differentiate these patients from patients with temporal lobe epilepsy or from patients with anxiety disorders. In this regard, a cut-off point of 70 was shown to yield a sensitivity of 75.5% and a specificity of 87.2%. Furthermore, the scale has a high internal consistency (Cronbach alpha and split half reliability of 0.89 and 0.92, respectively) (Sierra and Berrios, 2000). Recently, a German version of the CDS has been validated on 91 in-patients of a psychotherapy unit, 43 of whom had a DSM-IV diagnosis of depersonalization disorder (Michal *et al.*, 2004). In a related study (Michal *et al.*, 2005a) the performance of the CDS was compared with the dissociative experiences scale, and the depersonalization subscale of the German Narcissism Inventory on a sample of 144 psychotherapy patients with differing degrees of depersonalization (none = 51; mild = 45; moderate = 28; severe = 20). A comparison of ROC curves revealed that the areas under the curve and the rate of misclassification did not differ for the DES or the NI-DRP. The CDS, in turn, yielded the lower rate of misclassifications.

A Spanish (Molina Castillo *et al.*, 2006) and a Japanese (Sugiura *et al.*, 2008) version of the CDS have also been validated recently and found to have similar psychometric profiles to those reported above.

The Fewtrell Depersonalization Scale

The Fewtrell Depersonalization Scale (FDS) is a 35-item self-report questionnaire, covering four symptom domains: *derealization, depersonalization, desomatization* and *de-affectualization* (Fewtrell, 2000). Subjects are asked to indicate on a five-point scale the degree to which an item has been true, during the preceding month. The items are scored 0–4, resulting in a maximum score (for the most severe depersonalization) of 140; they include both negatively and positively biased items, e.g. a cut-off on the FDS-35 has previously been validated against a large normative sample and patients with personality disorders (Fewtrell, 2000). A recent study (Lambert *et al.*, 2001) used the Fewtrell scale to compare patients with depersonalization disorder and normal and clinical controls. It was found that the scale had a sensitivity of 85.7% and a specificity of 92.3% (i.e. 37 cases were identified correctly with three false-positives). Receiver operating characteristics (ROC) analysis yielded an area under the curve of 0.864. On the whole, this is a promising, fairly comprehensive scale, whose psychometric properties remain under-researched.

The Structured Clinical Interview for DSM-IV Dissociative Disorders (SCID-D)

This is a semi-structured interview, which evaluates five dissociative symptom domains: amnesia, depersonalization, derealization, identity confusion and identity alteration. It was designed to screen for, and diagnose, dissociative disorders as contained in DSM-IV (Steinberg, 1993; Steinberg *et al.*, 1993). It has been found to be a reliable and valid instrument, and has been used in recent studies to ascertain a diagnosis of depersonalization disorder. Given that it was designed to assess dissociation in general, its questions regarding depersonalization do not comprehensively assess the different symptom domains that constitute the condition.

The Structured Clinical Interview for Depersonalization–Derealization Spectrum (SCI-DER)

This is a new instrument designed to assess four symptom domains of depersonalization: (1) derealization; (2) somatopsychic depersonalization; (3) autopsychic depersonalization; and (4) affective depersonalization. The authors report excellent internal consistency (0.92), good test–retest reliability at 15–20 days ($r = 0.88$), and good convergent and discriminant validity (Mula *et al.*, 2008a, b). The scale is composed of a series of items, which are preceded by the question *"Have you ever experienced just for a few seconds or for days or months …?"*. The items themselves, which are to be answered in a 'yes' or 'no' dichotomous format, are mostly derived, with little or no modification from self-rating scales, such as the CDS and the DES. In this regard, given that the items are cast into a 'yes' or 'no' dichotomous format, this scale seems to have more the structure of a self-rating instrument than of a structured interview.

REFERENCES

Ackner, B. (1954). Depersonalisation I. Aetiology and phenomenology. *Journal of Mental Science*, **100**, 838–853.

Aderibigbe, Y. A., Bloch, R. M., Walker, W. R. (2001). Prevalence of depersonalization and derealization experiences in a rural population. *Social Psychiatry and Psychiatric Epidemiology*, **36**, 63–69.

American Psychiatric Association (APA) (1994). *Diagnostic and Statistical Manual of Mental Disorders. 4th edn.* Washington: DC, American Psychiatric Association.

Baker, D., Hunter E., Lawrence E. *et al.* (2003). Depersonalisation disorder: clinical features of 204 cases. *British Journal of Psychiatry*, **182**, 428–433.

Bliss, E. L., Clark, L. D., Charles, W. D. (1959). Study of sleep deprivation: Relationship to schizophrenia. *Archives of Neurology and Psychiatry*, **81**, 348–359.

Brauer, R., Harrow, M., Tucker, G. J. (1970). Depersonalization phenomena in psychiatric patients. *British Journal of Psychiatry*, **117**, 509–515.

Cappon, D. (1968). Fifty hours of wakefulness. *Psychophysiology*, **5**, 97–98.

Charbonneau, J., O'Connor, K. (1999). Depersonalization in a non-clinical sample. *Behavioural and Cognitive Psychotherapy*, **27**, 377–381.

Cohen, P., Cohen, J. (1984). The clinician's illusion. *Archives of General Psychiatry*, **41**, 1178–1182.

Cox, B. J., Swinson, R. P. (2002). Instrument to assess depersonalization-derealization in panic disorder. *Depression and Anxiety*, **15**, 172–175.

Dittrich, A. (1975). Comparison of altered states of consciousness induced by short-term sensory deprivation and trans-tetrahydrocannabinol. *Psychophysiology*, **22**, 547–560.

Dixon, J. C. (1963). Depersonalisation phenomena in a sample population of college students. *British Journal of Psychiatry*, **109**, 371–375.

Edwards, J. G., Angus, J. W. (1972). Depersonalization. *British Journal of Psychiatry*, **120**, 242–244.

Eggers, C. H. (1979). Depersonalisation und derealisation im Kindheit. *Praxis der Kinderpsychologie un Kinderpsychiatrie*, **28**, 231–236.

Elliot, G. C., Rosenberg M., Wagner, M. (1984). Transient depersonalization in youth. *Social Psychology Quarterly*, **47**, 115–129.

Fewtrell, W. D. (2000). *Fewtrell Depersonalisation Scale (FDS)*. Leicester: APT Press.

Horowitz, M. J. (1964). Depersonalization in spacemen and submariners. *Military Medicine*, **129**, 1058–1060.

Hunter, E. C., Phillips, M. L., Chalder, T., Sierra, M., David, A. S. (2003). Depersonalisation disorder: a cognitive-behavioural conceptualisation. *Behaviour Research and Therapy*, **41**, 1451–1467.

Hunter, E. C., Sierra, M., David, A. S. (2004). The epidemiology of depersonalisation and derealisation. A systematic review. *Social Psychiatry and Psychiatric Epidemiology*, **39**, 9–18.

Hunter, E. C., Baker, D., Phillips, M. L., Sierra, M., David, A. S. (2005). Cognitive-behaviour therapy for depersonalisation disorder: an open study. *Behaviour Research and Therapy*, **43**, 1121–1130.

Johnson, J. G., Cohen, P., Kasen, S., Brook, J. S. (2006). Dissociative disorders among adults in the community, impaired functioning, and axis I and II comorbidity. *Journal of Psychiatry Research*, **40**, 131–140.

Lambert, M. V., Senior, C., Fewtrell, W. D., Phillips, M. L., David, A. S. (2001). Primary and secondary depersonalisation disorder: a psychometric study. *Journal of Affective Disorders*, **63**, 249–256.

Leonard, K. N., Telch, M. J., Harrington, P. J. (1999). Dissociation in the laboratory: a comparison of strategies. *Behaviour Research and Therapy*, **37**, 49–61.

Meares, R., Grose, D. (1978). On depersonalization in adolescence: a consideration from the viewpoints on habituation and 'identity'. *British Journal of Medical Psychology*, **51**, 335–342.

Meyer, J. E. (1961). Depersonalisation in adolescence. *Psychiatry*, **24**, 357–360.

Michal, M., Sann, U., Niebecker, M. *et al.* (2004). Die Erfassung des Depersonalisation-Derealisations syndroms mit der deutschen Version der Cambridge Depersonalisation Scale (CDS). *Zeitschrift für Psychotherapie, Psychosomatik, Medizinische Psychologie*, **54**, 367–374.

Michal, M., Kaufhold, J., Engelbach, U. *et al.* (2005a). Zur Validität der Skala Derealisation/Depersonalisation des Narzissmusinventars. *Psychotherapie, Psychosomatik, Medizinische Psychologie*, **55**, 512–516.

Michal, M., Kaufhold, J., Grabhorn, R., Krakow, K., Overbeck, G., Heidenreich, T. (2005b). Depersonalization and social anxiety. *Journal of Nervous and Mental Diseases*, **193**, 629–632.

Michal, M., Beutel, M. E., Jordan, J., Zimmermann, M., Wolters, S., Heidenreich, T. (2007). Depersonalization, mindfulness, and childhood trauma. *Journal of Nervous and Mental Disease*, **195**, 693–696.

Michal, M., Wiltink, J., Subic-Wrana, C. *et al.* (2009). Prevalence, correlates and predictors of depersonalization experiences in the German general population. *Journal of Nervous and Mental Disease*, in press.

Molina Castillo, J. J., Martinez de la Iglesia, J., Albert Colomer, C., Berrios, G., Sierra, M., Luque, R. (2006). Cross-cultural adaptation and validation of the Cambridge Depersonalisation Scale. *Actas Españolas de Psiquiatría*, **34**, 185–192.

Moyano, O., Claudon, Ph. (2003). Expériences dissociatives sévères relevées dans un groupe d'étudiants français : à propos de la dépersonnalisation. *Annales Médico Psychologiques*, **161**, 183–189.

Mula, M., Pini, S., Lalugi, S. *et al.* (2008a). Validity and reliability of the Structured Clinical Interview for Depersonalization-Derealization Spectrum (SCI-DER). *Neuropsychiatric Disease and Treatment*, **4**, 977–984.

Mula, M., Pini, S., Preve, M., Masini, M., Giovannini, I., Cassano, G. B. (2008b). Clinical correlates of depersonalization symptoms in patients with bipolar disorder. *Journal of Affective Disorders*, **115**, 252–256.

Myers, D. H., Grant, G. A. (1972). Study of depersonalization in students. *British Journal of Psychiatry*, **121**, 59–65.

Office of Rare Diseases (ORD): http://rarediseases.info.nih.gov/. Accessed 2009.

Reed, G. F., Segman, G. (1964). Personality and depersonalization under sensory deprivation conditions. *Perceptual and Motor Skills*, **18**, 659–660.

Roberts, W. W. (1960). Normal and abnormal depersonalisation. *Journal of Mental Science*, **106**, 478–493.

Ross, C. A., Joshi, S., Currie, R. (1990). Dissociative experiences in the general population. *American Journal of Psychiatry*, **147**, 1547–1552.

Roth, M. (1998). Depersonalisation ser fahrungen bei Jugendlichen. *Zeitschrift Kinder Jugend psychiatrie und Psychotherapie*, **26**, 266–272.

Salfield, D. J. (1957). Autogenic training of a child with depersonalization. *Psychotherapie*, **2**, 232–235.

Salfield, D. J. (1958). Depersonalization and allied conditions in childhood. *Journal of Mental Science*, **134**, 470–472.

Schilder, P. (1935). *The Image and Appearance of the Human Body*. London: Kegan Paul.

Sedman, G. (1966). Depersonalization in a group of normal subjects. *British Journal of Psychiatry*, **112**, 907–912.

Shimizu, M., Sakamoto, S. (1986). Depersonalization in early adolescence. *Japanese Journal of Psychiatry and Neurology*, **40**, 603–608.

Shorvon, H. J. (1946). The depersonalisation syndrome. *Proceedings of the Royal Society of Medicine*, **39**, 779–792.

Sierra, M., Berrios, G. E. (2000). The Cambridge Depersonalization Scale: a new instrument for the measurement of depersonalization. *Psychiatry Research*, **93**, 153–164.

Sierra, M., Baker, D., Medford, N., David, A. S. (2005). Unpacking the depersonalization syndrome: an exploratory factor analysis on the Cambridge Depersonalization Scale. *Psychological Medicine*, **35**, 1523–1532.

Simeon, D. (2004). Depersonalisation disorder: a contemporary overview. *CNS Drugs*, **18**, 343–354.

Simeon, D., Knutelska, M. (2005). An open trial of naltrexone in the treatment of depersonalization disorder. *Journal of Clinical Psychopharmacology*, **25**, 267–270.

Simeon, D., Guralnik, O., Gross, S., Stein, D. J., Schmeidler, J., Hollander, E. (1998). The detection and measurement of depersonalization disorder. *Journal of Nervous and Mental Disease*, **186**, 536–542.

Simeon, D., Guralnik, O., Schmeidler, J. (2001a). Development of a depersonalization severity scale. *Journal of Trauma and Stress*, **14**, 341–349.

Simeon, D., Guralnik, O., Schmeidler, J., Sirof, B., Knutelska, M. (2001b). The role of childhood interpersonal trauma in depersonalization disorder. *American Journal of Psychiatry*, **158**, 1027–1033.

Simeon, D., Guralnik, O., Knutelska, M., Schmeidler, J. (2002). Personality factors associated with dissociation: temperament, defenses, and cognitive schemata. *American Journal of Psychiatry*, **159**, 489–491.

Simeon, D., Knutelska, M., Nelson, D., Guralnik, O. (2003a). Feeling unreal: a depersonalization disorder update of 117 cases. *Journal of Clinical Psychiatry*, **64**, 990–997.

Simeon, D., Nelson, D., Elias, R., Greenberg, J., Hollander, E. (2003b). Relationship of personality to dissociation and childhood trauma in borderline personality disorder. *CNS Spectrum*, **8**, 755–762.

Simeon, D., Kozin, D. S., Segal, K., Lerch, B., Dujour, R., Giesbrecht, T. (2008). De-constructing depersonalization: further evidence for symptom clusters. *Psychiatry Research*, **157**, 303–306.

Steinberg, M. (1991). The spectrum of depersonalization: assessment and treatment. In Tasman, A., Goldfinger, S. M. (eds.). *APA Review of Psychiatry*, **10**, 223–247.

Steinberg, M. (1993). *Structured Clinical Interview for DSM-IV Dissociative Disorders (SCID-D)*. 3rd edn. Washington, DC: American Psychiatric Press.

Steinberg, M. (1995). *Handbook for the Assessment of Dissociation. A Clinical Guide*. Washington, DC: American Psychiatric Press.

Steinberg, M., Rounsaville, B., Cicchetti, D. (1991). Detection of dissociative disorders in psychiatric patients by a screening instrument and a structured diagnostic interview. *American Journal of Psychiatry*, **148**, 1050–1054.

Stewart, W. A. (1964). Panel on depersonalization. *Journal of the American Psychoanalytic Association*, **12**, 171–186.

Sugiura, M., Hirowawa, M., Nishi, Y., Yamada, Y., Mizuno, M., Tanaka, S. (2008). Development of a Japanese version of the Cambridge Depersonalization Scale and application to Japanese University Students. Annual Reports of Juntendo Institute of Mental Health, 93–101 (no issue number stated).

Toglia, M. P., Neuschatz, J. S., Goodwin, K. A. (1999). Recall accuracy and illusory memories: when more is less. *Memory*, **7**, 233–256.

Trueman, D. (1984a). Depersonalization in a nonclinical population. *Journal of Psychology*, **116**, 107–112.

Trueman, D. (1984b). Depersonalization in a college sample. *Journal of General Psychology*, **14**, 980–989.

Trueman, D. (1984). Anxiety and depersonalization and derealization experiences. *Psychological Reports*, **54**, 91–96.

World Health Organization (1992). F48.1. Depersonalisation-derealisation syndrome. In *The ICD-10 Classification of Mental and Behavioural Disorders. Clinical Descriptions and Diagnostic Guidelines*. Geneva: World Health Organization. pp. 171–173.

4

'Drug-induced' depersonalization disorder

Introduction

As will be described in Chapter 8, it has been established that cannabis and other drugs can reliably induce depersonalization in a dose-dependent manner and under placebo control situations. In such circumstances the duration of the depersonalization experience is time-locked to the duration of the intoxication. A more intriguing and difficult to explain phenomenon, however, is the apparent development of prolonged and persistent depersonalization after a single or limited exposure to cannabis (Moran, 1986; Berkowitz, 1981; Keshaven and Lishman, 1986), or other drugs such as hallucinogenics, ecstasy or ketamine (Medford *et al.*, 2003; Simeon *et al.*, 2009). In most of these cases patients consider their chronic symptoms to be identical to those experienced during the acute intoxication state (Szymanski, 1981). Although it is common for some patients to have previously used cannabis with no adverse effects, they typically remember the triggering intoxication episode as a terrifying or life-threatening experience accompanied by a feeling of loss of control (Moran, 1986). In a recent study of 196 cases of 'drug-induced' depersonalization, the large majority of participants acknowledged such an experience of 'bad trip' preceding the onset of depersonalization (Simeon *et al.*, 2009). 'Bad trips' have been shown to occur at times of exposure to psychosocial stress or distressing life events (Szymansky, 1981), and seem to be followed by severe anticipatory anxiety, panic attacks and agoraphobia (Moran, 1986). Suggestive of the highly aversive and frightening nature of the experience, Simeon *et al.* (2009) found that 'the majority of individuals do not experiment with the culprit drug ever again'. It is plausible that such high levels of anticipatory anxiety and avoidance play a role in the maintenance of ensuing depersonalization feelings.

Although in some cases the state of intoxication seems to lead seamlessly to persistent depersonalization, more commonly its onset occurs after a 'sober' period of time, which can go from a few hours to several days. The following case illustrates this.

A 25-year-old woman, with no previous medical or psychiatric history, claimed that her symptoms started whist on holiday with her boyfriend when she tried a 'cannabis cake'. For several hours she found herself in an altered state of consciousness accompanied by a most agonizing feeling of depersonalization. Although she felt fine for most of the following week, over the following days she went on to have occasional transient and terrifying experiences, when she would claim to experience an almost identical replica of the symptoms she had whilst intoxicated. Such intermittent episodes went on for approximately 2 months until one day the condition became constant: "it felt as if I had no legs, like numb. I also had the strange feeling that my self was at my side or behind me." After 1 year and a half of experiencing these symptoms constantly, she made a gradual recovery with the aid of pharmacological treatment.

Given that cannabis is known to be excreted over several weeks, the occurrence of symptoms spanning months or years following drug usage begs for an explanation. While some authors have proposed the possibility of residual neurotoxic effects, or the existence of a protracted cannabis withdrawal syndrome (Keshaven and Lishman, 1986), others have favoured psychological explanations (Szymansky, 1981; Moran, 1986). Thus, for Szymansky it is likely that once "the patients had experienced depersonalization, intrapsychic factors may have contributed to its continued used as a defence mechanism after acute intoxication" (Szymansky, 1981, p. 232). In fact, it was further suggested that some of these cases could be conceptualized as a kind of conversion disorder "that manifested itself through psychological rather than physical symptoms" (Berkowitz, 1981).

Some of the clinical features of 'drug-induced' persistent depersonalization are redolent of 'flashback' experiences (Keshaven and Lishman, 1986). The term 'flashback' was originally used in relation to LSD usage (Sierra and Berrios, 1997), but was subsequently extended to describe the effects of other drugs such as ketamine and cannabis and in the last two decades in relation to psychological trauma. A 'flashback' was defined as a "sudden re-experience of images, feelings, or sensations originally associated with drug use which may have occurred weeks or months earlier" (McGee, 1984, p. 273). Indeed, it is known that the phenomenology of such recurrent episodes can encompass a vast range of experiences, which may include "distortions of time sense, self-image, or reality sense" (Horowitz, 1969). For example, one study found that, in 34 LSD-related psychiatric admissions, 32% of patients admitted to experiences of "spontaneous return of perceptual distortions or feelings of depersonalization similar to those experienced under the influence of LSD" (Robbins et al., 1967). Another study found that 55% of hallucinogen users in the community reported 'flashback' experiences. Listed as the most frequent were recurrent episodes of depersonalization, disorientation, and the spontaneous appearance of colour hazes or curtains (Barron et al., 1970).

In view of the intriguing overlaps between drug induced 'flashbacks' and 'drug-induced' depersonalization, the idea that the former may shed light on the origin and nature of the latter is worth while exploring. A brief overview on the predisposing factors which can lead to 'flashbacks' suggests that they are indeed relevant to drug-induced depersonalization (Lerner *et al.*, 2002).

Although initial theories of drug-induced flashbacks favoured biological explanations such as the late release of tissue-stored drug molecules, or the development of seizure-like activity (i.e. kindling), there is no convincing evidence supporting such views (McGee, 1984). In fact, the following number of observations suggest instead that 'flashbacks' are psychologically mediated to a large extent and support the idea that 'drug-induced' depersonalization might be conceptualized as a type of 'flashback' phenomenon. In fact, it is worth noticing that most of the following predisposing factors to 'flashbacks' have also been described in relation to depersonalization experiences.

(1) Flashbacks are frequently reported to start occurring following a distressing episode of drug intoxication (i.e. 'bad trip') characterized by intense anxiety (Saidel and Babineau, 1976). In this regard, it would seem that the sole exposure to the drug is not sufficient, and many subjects who have used drugs for years without ever experiencing untoward psychological effects go on to develop flashbacks after a dysphoric experience (Juve, 1972).

(2) Physiological stress and fatigue often precede the onset of flashbacks (Horowitz, 1969).

(3) People with premorbid obsessional personalities seem at risk for the development of 'flashbacks' (Saidel and Babineau, 1976).

(4) Flashbacks can be induced through suggestion, even in drug users with no history of the phenomenon (Heaton, 1975). In fact, some people are able to self-induce the experience just by thinking about it. It is of interest that people with a history of drug-induced flashbacks have been shown to score higher on hypnotizability measures (Fischer, 1976), and seem predisposed to become absorbed in role playing situations (Matefy, 1980).

In view of the above observations, some authors have suggested that 'flashbacks' are manifestations of a 'state-dependent' learning process (McGee, 1984). In this regard, flashbacks might correspond to sensory, implicit memories whose retrieval takes the form of an actual re-experiencing of the original altered state of consciousness, not unlike the way in which amputees with phantom pains often re-experience the exact quality of previously experienced pains before the amputation (Sierra and Berrios, 1999). One study found that up to 57% of subjects experiencing flashbacks rated them as 'exact' phenomenological replicas of previous drug experiences (Shick *et al.*, 1970 and Matefy *et al.*, 1978). For example, one researcher reported the case of a psychiatrist who had previously enjoyed the regular use of cannabis for its relaxing effects, until he had an extremely distressing experience whilst experimenting with LSD (Weil, 1970). Following this incident, he noticed that any attempt to smoke cannabis would cause him to re-experience a replica of his LSD intoxication. A similar case seen by the author was that of a young male with depersonalization disorder, whose symptoms had started in the context of cannabis smoking. After having made a gradual recovery, he had a sudden severe relapse, after taking a puff from a friend's cigarette. Given that he had stopped smoking since the onset of depersonalization, it would seem that the act of taking a cigarette to his mouth was enough to cue a flashback experience of the initial incident. His symptoms continued unabated for a week and then gradually subsided. The sensory experiential retrieval of events has been well documented in a range of psychiatric and neurological conditions (Sierra and Berrios, 1999). Consistent with this observation, a survey on 196 'drug-induced' chronic depersonalizations revealed that, if subjects try the drug again, it reliably has the effect of rekindling the intensity of the condition (Simeon et al., 2009).

A similar cueing effect has been observed by recalling a previous depersonalization event while under the effects of drugs. For example, a patient seen by the author related that, at the age of 18, he experienced a full-blown episode of depersonalization whilst under the effects of LSD. Unfortunately the depersonalization did not subside as he sobered up and, in fact, remained unabated for the next 15 months, after which it gradually subsided. He remained symptom free for the next 6 years and, during this time, he did not use any drugs. He then tried cannabis at a party and, at the beginning, did not experience any untoward effects. However, as he was talking to some friends, the conversation turned to his previous experience of depersonalization, and as he found himself struggling to convey what the experience had felt like, he suddenly found himself sliding back into it. He described the experience as being identical to the one he had first experienced under LSD: "It feels as if I am not here, I see the world as on a TV screen; the sound of my voice sounds very strange, as if it did not come from me"; he also found his reflection in the mirror as unrelated to him. This second experience remained constant and had been so for more than a year and a half at the time of assessment.

In keeping with the above observations, it has been found that memories of strongly emotional or traumatic events have a very strong implicit, perceptual component (Ehlers et al., 2004).

One recent study found that, in a series of 164 consecutive cases of depersonalization disorder referred to a depersonalization clinic, 40 attributed the onset of the condition to an episode of illicit drug usage. Most patients claimed that symptoms of depersonalization started during the period of intoxication or within 72 hours of ingesting the drug. Twenty attributed the onset of their symptoms to cannabis, either on its own or in combination with other drugs. Four attributed the onset to 'Ecstasy' (MDMA), two to LSD and one to ketamine (Medford et al., 2003). A similar drug list was reported in another cohort of depersonalization disorder patients, who ascribed the onset of depersonalization disorder to drug usage (Simeon et al., 2003).

A comparison of the 40 'drug-induced depersonalization' disorder cases with 122 non-drug induced cases revealed that the phenomenology of depersonalization across the two groups was strikingly similar, hence suggesting that drug-induced depersonalization does not appear to represent a distinct clinical syndrome. However, whilst 90% of those in the drug-induced group admitted to a history of anxiety and/or panic attacks, only 29% in the non-drug group did (Medford *et al.*, 2003). This suggests that anxiety may be a mediating factor in the origin of 'drug-induced' cases.

Another study compared 196 drug-induced chronic depersonalization cases with 198 non-drug-induced counterparts and found an absence of significant differences in regards to phenomenology, illness course, impairment levels, suicidality and treatment response (Simeon *et al.*, 2009). In keeping with previous studies, the two most common precipitating drugs were cannabis and hallucinogens, followed by ecstasy and ketamine.

To sum up, various studies support the view that an interplay between anxiety and 'flashback-like' experiences may play an important role in the establishment of chronic depersonalization following the use of drugs. It seems plausible to think that, in a subgroup of particularly anxious patients, the experience of a 'bad trip' can acquire traumatic proportions, so that the ensuing anxiety, together with feelings of not being in control, may trigger depersonalization symptoms. Unfortunately, the latter can only amplify the sense of terror and lack of control, hence setting in motion a vicious circle which can potentially sustain the symptoms in time. The other component of this self-perpetuating mechanism is represented by an intense anticipatory anxiety, avoidance behaviour, and the ability of sensory or cognitive cues associated with the original experience to trigger a 'flashback' re-experiencing of the 'bad trip' and ensuing depersonalization. It remains to be seen if the adoption of such a model, which views the development of drug-induced depersonalization along the lines of a 'post-traumatic condition', can be useful in furthering the understanding and treatment of this baffling condition.

REFERENCES

Barron, S. P., Lowinger, P., Ebner, E. (1970). A clinical examination of chronic LSD use in the community. *Comprehensive Psychiatry*, **11**, 69–79.

Berkowitz, H. L. (1981). Marijuana-induced depersonalization. *American Journal of Psychiatry*, **138**, 1396.

Ehlers, A., Hackmann, A., Michael, T. (2004). Intrusive re-experiencing in post-traumatic stress disorder: phenomenology, theory, and therapy. *Memory*, **12**, 403–415.

Fischer, R. (1976). Hypnotic recall and flashback: the remembrance of things present. *Confinia Psychiatrica*, **19**, 149–173.

Heaton, R. K. (1975). Subject expectancy and environmental factors as determinants of psychedelic flashback experiences. *The Journal of Nervous and Mental Disease*, **161**, 157–165.

Horowitz, M. J. (1969). Flashbacks: recurrent intrusive images after the use of LSD. *American Journal of Psychiatry*, **126**, 565–569.

Juve, J. L. (1972). Bad drug trips and flashbacks. *Child Welfare*, **51**, 41–50.

Keshaven, M. S., Lishman, W. A. (1986). Prolonged depersonalization following cannabis abuse. *British Journal of Addiction*, **81**, 140–142.

Lerner, A. G., Gelkopf, M., Skladman, I. *et al.* (2002). Flashback and hallucinogen persisting perception disorder: clinical aspects and pharmacological treatment approach. *The Israel Journal of Psychiatry and Related Sciences*, **39**, 92–99.

Matefy, R. (1980). Role-play theory of psychedelic drug flashbacks. *Journal of Consulting and Clinical Psychology*, **48**, 551–553.

Matefy, R. E., Hayes, C., Hirsch, J. (1978). Psychedelic drug flashbacks: subjective reports and biographical data. *Addictive Behavior*, **3**, 165–178.

McGee, R. (1984). Flashbacks and memory phenomena. A comment on "Flashback phenomena – clinical and diagnostic dilemmas". *Journal of Nervous and Mental Diseases*, **172**, 273–278.

Medford, N., Baker, D., Hunter, E. *et al.* (2003). Chronic depersonalization following illicit drug use: a controlled analysis of 40 cases. *Addiction*, **98**, 1731–1736.

Moran, C. (1986). Depersonalisation and agoraphobia associated with marihuana use. *British Journal of Medical Psychology*, **59**, 187–196.

Robbins, E., Frosch, W. A., Stern, M. (1967). Further observations on untoward reactions to LSD. *American Journal of Psychiatry*, **124**, 393–395.

Saidel, D. R., Babineau, R. (1976). Prolonged LSD flashbacks as conversion reactions. *Journal of Nervous and Mental Diseases*, **163**, 352–355.

Sierra, M., Berrios, G. E. (1999). Flashbulb memories and other repetitive images: a psychiatric perspective. *Comprehensive Psychiatry*, **40**, 115–125.

Shick, J. F. E., Smith, D. E. (1970). Analysis of the LSD flashback. *Journal of Psychedelic Drugs*, **3**, 13–19.

Simeon, D., Knutelska, M., Nelson, D., Guralnik, O. (2003). Feeling unreal: a depersonalization disorder update of 117 cases. *Journal of Clinical Psychiatry*, **64**, 990–997.

Simeon, D., Kozin, D., Segal, K., Lerch, B. (2009). Is depersonalization disorder initiated by drug use any different? A survey of 394 adults. *Journal of Clinical Psychiatry*, in press.

Szymanski, H. V. (1981). Prolongued depersonalisation after marihuana use. *American Journal of Psychiatry*, **138**, 231–233.

Weil, A. T. (1970). Adverse reactions to marihuana. Classification and suggested treatment. *New England Journal of Medicine*, **282**, 997–1000.

5

Psychiatric comorbidity
of depersonalization

Introduction

Studies carried out on psychiatric patients with a whole variety of diagnoses show that, as a comorbid phenomenon, depersonalization is highly prevalent (Hunter *et al.*, 2004). For example, 80% of 212 psychiatric in-patients admitted to present or past depersonalization experiences, although in only 12% was depersonalization severe and lasting (Brauer *et al.*, 1970). Another study found that 40% of 100 psychiatric in-patients endorsed at least five features of depersonalization (Noyes *et al.*, 1977). Interestingly, the presence of anxiety was found to be significantly associated with depersonalization. More recently, researchers have found a similarly high prevalence (Michal *et al.*, 2005) using validated measures of depersonalization such as the structured interview for DSM-IV dissociative disorders (Steinberg *et al.*, 1990) and the Cambridge Depersonalization Scale (Sierra and Berrios, 2000). The study comprised 143 first admission in-patients of a clinic specialized in psychosomatic conditions. The authors found a 1-month prevalence of ICD-10, 'Depersonalization-derealization syndrome' (WHO, 1992) to be 23.1% (*n* = 33). In keeping with the above studies, a total of 62.9% reported depersonalization symptoms, regardless of severity. Moreover, the group with pathological depersonalization was characterized by a high comorbidity with anxiety disorders and had higher levels of impairment.

Although it has been found that depersonalization can indeed co-occur with virtually any psychiatric condition, patterns of comorbidity clearly show that only a few conditions seem particularly predisposed to be accompanied by severe depersonalization (Hunter *et al.*, 2004).

The detection and diagnosis of depersonalization, even when it seems secondary to another condition, is important for several reasons:
(1) Depersonalization is a significant source of distress and impairment in its own right and its neglect in clinical discussions with patients often leads to the establishment of a poor doctor–patient relationship and to non-compliance with treatment.

(2) Increasing evidence suggests that the presence of comorbid depersonalization has an effect on the clinical manifestations of the comorbid condition and can be a marker of severity and poor prognosis (Mula *et al.*, 2007).

(3) There is emerging evidence that, regardless of comorbidity, depersonalization often responds to a number of medications, some of which are not conventionally used in psychiatry (Sierra, 2008).

What follows is a review of the main comorbid conditions and the nature of their associations with depersonalization.

Acute-stress related depersonalization

It has been fairly well established that in the face of life-threatening situations people often experience depersonalization (Mayer-Gross *et al.*, 1969; Noyes and Kletti, 1977). This suggests that acute, overwhelming anxiety can act as a powerful trigger of such episodes. In a retrospective study of accident survivors, it was found that 66% of participants remembered having experienced depersonalization at the time of the accident (Noyes and Kletti, 1977). In recent years, similar findings have been reported in victims of natural disasters or violent attacks and confirm the view that depersonalization, as a transient experience, is a commonplace occurrence in a significant proportion of victims (Wilkinson, 1983). For example, in a study of survivors of the San Francisco Bay Area earthquake, it was found that 25% of a sample of normal students admitted to marked depersonalization during and immediately after the earthquake, and 40% described derealization (Cardena and Spiegel, 1993). Likewise, 54% of the survivors of an airline crash-landing acknowledged derealization symptoms (Sloan, 1988). Research on hostage-taking situations has also shown that more than half of the victims have experienced feelings of unreality, lack of agency feelings and emotional numbing (Hillman, 1981).

Two different explanations have been advanced to explain the high prevalence of depersonalization during life-threatening situations. One of them suggests that depersonalization represents a useful functional response elicited by high levels of anxiety and feelings of not being in control. According to this view, depersonalization could be seen as a 'hard-wired' response, which possibly evolved to ensure the preservation of adaptive behaviour during situations likely to elicit overwhelming and potentially disorganizing anxiety. In contrast to the 'fight or flight' response, depersonalization would normally be triggered by perceived life-threatening situations in which the individual does not seem to have control over the situation, or when the source of danger cannot be localized in external space (e.g. earthquake; car crash, etc.). In such circumstances depersonalization will generate a state of emotional disengagement whilst preserving a state of vigilant alertness (Sierra and Berrios, 1998). From a different stance, psychoanalysts also have long endorsed the view and that depersonalization operates as a defence mechanism against intra-psychic conflicts (Federn, 1926; Feigenbaum, 1937; Oberndorf, 1935, 1950). Some support for the 'protective' view of depersonalization has been marshalled by experimental findings, which show that patients with depersonalization disorder show anomalous neural responses, which are selective to emotional pictures with disgusting or fear eliciting contents (Phillips and Sierra, 2003). From a more clinical stance, other researchers carried out a study on 75 victims of traumatic events in order to examine the relationship between the occurrence of depersonalization during a traumatic event and the emergence of subsequent psychiatric symptomatology (Shilony and Grossman, 1993). As predicted by the 'protective response theory' of depersonalization, those participants who had experienced depersonalization were found to show significantly less psychopathology at the time of study, as compared with those who did not experience depersonalization.

A second view of depersonalization, which has its origins in Janet's views of dissociation, contends that the condition results from a disruption in conscious experience brought about by trauma or extreme anxiety. According to this view, depersonalization is a non-specific, dysfunctional dissociative state devoid of any protective function. Terms such as 'peritraumatic dissociation' (Marmar *et al.*, 1994) or 'acute stress disorder' (Spiegel *et al.*, 2000) have been used recently to describe acute dissociative responses to trauma whose symptoms overlap to some extent with those of depersonalization. For example, peritraumatic dissociation "… may take the form of altered time sense … profound feelings of unreality… experiences of depersonalization; out-of-body experiences; altered pain perception; altered body image or feelings of disconnection from one's body" amongst others (Marmar *et al.*, 1994). 'Acute stress disorder' in turn, has been described as the occurrence of three (or more) of the following dissociative symptoms during or after experiencing the traumatic event (Zoellner *et al.*, 2003): a subjective sense of numbing, detachment or absence of emotional responsiveness. A reduction in awareness of his or her surroundings (e.g. 'being in a daze'); and depersonalization–dissociative amnesia (i.e. inability to recall an important aspect of the trauma).

Contrary to the study discussed above, which suggested a protective role of depersonalization (Shilony and Grossman, 1993), it has been found that the presence of acute dissociation during trauma predicts the subsequent emergence of psychopathology (Taal and Faber, 1997). In particular, a prevailing view has emerged in the last decade, which views the occurrence of 'peritraumatic dissociation' as a risk factor for the later development of 'post-traumatic stress disorder' (PTSD). A recent meta-analysis, which included 35 empirical studies, found 'peritraumatic dissociation' to be a moderate risk factor for PTSD (Breh and Seidler, 2007). In the same vein, growing evidence suggests that ketamine, which induces transient dissociative states and cognitive dysfunction, can aggravate early post-traumatic stress reactions when administered in the acute trauma phase (Schönenberg *et al.*, 2005, 2008). Such findings would seem to suggest that dissociation disables rather than enables adaptation to traumatic situations. However, one potential conceptual flaw stems from the unwarranted assumption that acute dissociation and PTSD are completely independent constructs (Breh and Seidler, 2007). In fact, since the concept of 'peritraumatic dissociation' overlaps to some extent with PTSD (e.g. it has been considered as an acute version of PTSD), correlations between the two are to be expected. It may be that, rather than there being a causal relationship between the two, it is the intensity of the perceived trauma which predisposes to both. For example, one study found that, amongst 85 female victims of recent rape (Griffin *et al.*, 1997), those who had severe 'peritraumatic dissociation' were those who had a higher perception of life threat during the rape. In view of this, the authors espoused a defensive view of dissociation and suggested that 'peritraumatic dissociation' must have acted as a mechanism used to deal with extreme anxiety.

Unfortunately, most studies on 'peritraumatic dissociation' have focused on its relationship with PTSD, and have thereby neglected any potential effects on other forms of psychopathology. Moreover, given that both peritraumatic dissociation and acute stress response include other dissociative symptoms in addition to depersonalization, it might still be the case that symptoms such as confusion and amnesia may obscure any protective effect of depersonalization. In fact, in the study, which found a protective effect of depersonalization on psychopathology, patients exhibiting other dissociative symptoms such as amnesia were excluded (Shilony and Grossman, 1993).

Anxiety disorders and depersonalization

The association between depersonalization and chronic anxiety disorders has been known since the early descriptions of depersonalization by Krishaber (1873). Indeed, most of the patients complaining of 'feelings of unreality' described in his *Névropathie Cérébro-Cardiaque* suffered from episodes of paroxysmal anxiety quite reminiscent of panic attacks. During the mid twentieth century Roth (1959) coined the term 'phobic anxiety depersonalization syndrome' to refer to cases in which the association was particularly apparent. Such a close relationship between depersonalization and anxiety has been found to be present all along the depersonalization spectrum. Thus, a significant correlation between anxiety and depersonalization has been found in non-clinical populations (Trueman, 1984); in psychiatric in-patients regardless of primary diagnosis (Noyes *et al.*, 1977); and in patients with depersonalization disorder (Baker *et al.*, 2003; Simeon *et al.*, 2003b). In fact, of all emotional states, anxiety was found to be the strongest predictor of depersonalization (Simeon *et al.*, 2003b).

Subsequent studies have emphasized the role of panic, as it has been found that the prevalence of depersonalization is much higher in panic disorder than in generalized anxiety (Noyes *et al.*, 1992). Recent findings suggest that the experience of panic can indeed be a mediating mechanism capable of triggering depersonalization responses during stressful or traumatic situations (Bryant and Panasetis, 2005; Nixon *et al.*, 2004). It has also been suggested that panic-like episodes mediate experiences of depersonalization associated with the use of illicit drugs (Medford *et al.*, 2003).

The association between depersonalization and panic spans along a continuum of severity. At one end, we find patients who experience transient depersonalization only during panic attacks. In some patients, however, depersonalization outlasts the latter and is present between attacks. At the other end of the spectrum, patients experience continuous depersonalization, even after complete remission of recurrent panic attacks.

Depersonalization as a symptom of panic attacks

The frequency of depersonalization amongst patients with panic disorder has been estimated to be around 50% in most Western countries (Swinson and Kuch, 1990). Interestingly, it has been found that, as compared with panic patients who don't depersonalize during panic attacks, those who do have an earlier onset of panic (Segui *et al.*, 2000; Ball *et al.*, 1997; Cassano *et al.*, 1989; Katerndahl and Talamantes, 2000), a more severe course (i.e. greater number of attacks, worse level of functioning), higher prevalence of agoraphobia and illness phobia (Benedetti *et al.*, 1997; Segui *et al.*, 2000) and show more atypical clinical features and abnormal EEG (Edlund *et al.*, 1987). For example, one study reported temporal lobe electroencephalographic abnormalities in panic disorder patients with depersonalization as compared with those with panic disorder without depersonalization (Locatelli *et al.*, 1993). In particular, patients with depersonalization showed increased slow activity and bilateral lack of fast alpha frequency response to odour stimulation. The validity of this finding is uncertain, however, as the same researchers were unable to replicate it (Locatelli *et al.*, 1995). Research into what predisposes some panic disorder patients to depersonalize during panic attacks has not been conclusive. One study found that, although 69% of patients with panic disorder experienced depersonalization or derealization during their panic attacks, panic disorder patients were no more likely to experience dissociative experiences as assessed by the Dissociative Experience Scale than patients with other anxiety disorders (Ball *et al.*, 1997). Likewise, other researchers found no evidence in support of their hypothesized association between depersonalization during panic attacks and a history of childhood trauma (Marshall *et al.*, 2000). More recently, however, another research group re-examined the latter hypothesis in a sample of 186 adults extracted from the National Comorbidity Survey, who met DSM-III-R criteria for panic disorder (Lachlan *et al.*, 2001). As compared with the nondepersonalization group, the depersonalization group reported more frequently a history of serious neglect as a child (13.8%, versus 3.9%, respectively), as well as a history of rape before age 16 (11%, versus 1.3%). Interestingly, no differences in regards to childhood abuse were found for any of the other symptoms of a panic attack. Such findings are in agreement with recent studies showing that a history of childhood neglect predicts the development of depersonalization symptoms (Michal *et al.*, 2007) or depersonalization disorder (Simeon *et al.*, 2001).

Comorbidity of depersonalization disorder and panic disorder

As described above, some patients in whom initial episodes of depersonalization are circumscribed to panic attacks go on to experience long-lasting episodes or continuous depersonalization, which no longer seems dependent on panic. In fact, it is not uncommon for constant depersonalization to remain unabated after panic attacks have been successfully treated (Hollander *et al.*, 1989). In their series of 117 cases of depersonalization disorder, Simeon *et al.* (2003a) found that, while the lifetime prevalence of panic disorder was 30.8%, only 12% had the condition at the time of the study. This would seem to support the view that recurrent panic attacks are frequent at the beginning of depersonalization disorder, but tend to subside after the condition becomes established.

Depersonalization and social anxiety

Paul Schilder (1938) was perhaps one of the first to draw attention to a close relationship between depersonalization experiences and what he termed as social neurosis. It has indeed now become well established that complaints of distress in social situations and resulting avoidance are commonplace in patients with depersonalization disorder (Simeon *et al.*, 2003b; Michal *et al.*, 2006); and a significant correlation has been found between measures of depersonalization and social anxiety in both clinical and non-clinical populations (Michal *et al.*, 2005). Such a relationship is not surprising, given that both social phobia and depersonalization are characterized by heightened self-observation and self-monitoring. For example, scores on items describing social situations such as: *"I can suddenly become aware of my own voice and of others listening to me"* or *"I feel tense if I am alone with just one other person"* have been found to predict global scores on the Cambridge Depersonalization Scale (Michal *et al.*, 2005).

Recent studies on large cohorts of patients with depersonalization disorder have found a high comorbidity with social anxiety. For example, one such study found that 30% of 117 patients met criteria for social phobia and 23% for avoidant personality disorder (Simeon *et al.*, 2003a). Strikingly similar results were obtained by other researchers, who compared 45 patients with patho-logical depersonalization with 55 patients with mild or no depersonalization (Michal *et al.*, 2006). It was found that whilst the prevalence of social phobia was 29% in those with pathological depersonalization, it was only 5% in the comparison group.

Mood disorders and depersonalization

An association between depression and depersonalization has been known for a long time. As early as 1880, Shäfer (1880; p. 242) drew attention to a form of depression attended by 'feelings of unreality' and striking emotional numbing. Shäfer spoused Griessinger's views that depersonalization (not called so by him) was mainly characterized by a profound emotional numbing and coined the term *Melancolia Anaesthetica* to describe the condition on the assumption that it was related to depression. This view was subsequently endorsed by writers such as Kraepelin (1896) and Juliusburger (1912) and the assumption was made that depersonalization was either a pathognomonic manifestation of depression or a subtype of affective psychosis. Lewis (1934), in his review on the phenomenology of depression, also wrote extensively on the association between depression and depersonalization, and went as far as to suggest that depressive anhedonia and depersonalization might be two different ways to describe the same phenomenon. Such a view was soon criticized on the grounds that depersonalization had distinct phenomenological features, which clearly set it aside from depression as a syndrome in its own right (Shorvon, 1946). In spite of this, the fact remains that there is a moderate comorbidity of deperson-alization symptoms and major depression. For example, as early as 1935, Mayer-Gross reported that 50% of his patients with chronic depersonalization described the onset of their symptoms during the course of an episode of depression (Mayer-Gross, 1935). However, as depersonalization becomes fully manifested, its relationship with depression is no longer clear, and the condition seems to follow an independent course. In fact, Mayer-Gross thought the actual comorbidity between depression and chronic depersonalization to be low: "Depersonalization occurs in only a small minority (10%–12%) of the patients with depressive illness and is generally confined to the complaint of blunting or deadness of feeling, which is the least specific part of the deperson-alization syndrome. When depersonalization is prominent and presents in its complete form, the diagnosis of depression requires careful reconsideration ... it is with the affect of anxiety and not with depression that depersonalization is most closely associated" (Mayer-Gross and Slater, 1969 p. 122). In their study on 117 patients with depersonalization disorder, Simeon *et al.* (2003a) found that, whilst the lifetime prevalence of major depression was 66.7%, its prevalence at the time of the study was only 10.3%. Moreover, a recent study comparing a sample of 45 patients with pathological depersonalization (ICD-10 depersonalization-derealization syndrome) with 55 patients with mild or no depersonalization, did not find any significant difference in the prevalence of depression between the two groups, which suggests that the association between depersonalization and depression is non-specific (Michal *et al.*, 2006).

A recent study on 1073 depressed in-patients found that 30.9% endorsed the depersonalization item of the Hamilton Depression Scale. It was found that, in those with a diagnosis of atypical depression, the prevalence of depersonalization rose to 52%, while it was 27% in those with typical depressive features (Seemüller *et al.*, 2008). Interestingly, in another study comparing 44 patients with affective disorders, it was found that, even when euthymic or mildly symptomatic, 18% and 14% admitted to derealization and depersonalization experiences, respectively. Such figures were found comparable with those of patients with temporal lobe epilepsy, but significantly higher than those found in controls with chronic hypertension (Silberman *et al.*, 1985). Similarly, depersonalization was reported by 17.6% of 51 patients with bipolar mood disorder (Ali *et al.*, 1997). It would seem that depersonalization symptoms are more frequent in patients with an early onset of bipolar mood disorder, while derealization is more prevalent in those bipolar patients with comorbid panic attacks (Mula *et al.*, 2008). It would seem, however, that depersonalization episodes have not been observed during manic states (Steinberg, 1991). In fact, cases of chronic depersonalization have been reported, where the remission of symptoms following treatment with benzodiazepines coincides with the emergence of an acute manic state (Liebowitz *et al.*, 1980; Bourgeois *et al.*, 1986).

Several early writers on depersonalization (Mayer-Gross, 1935; Saperstein, 1949; Ackner, 1954) made the intriguing observation that, in patients with depression who also experience depersonalization, the latter tends to be present only in the early stages of depression and that, in cases of psychotic depression, feelings of unreality apparently give way to the development of nihilistic or hypochondriac delusional ideas, as if the ineffable experience of depersonalization becomes transformed into a delusion (Young *et al.*, 1994). In order to test this hypothesis, Glitteson (1967) predicted that deluded depressives would exhibit a lower incidence of depersonalization as compared with non-deluded depressive patients. His retrospective analysis of 398 cases of depressive psychosis failed to show any significant difference between the two groups. Thus, depersonalization was present in 14% of those deluded and in 17% of those non-deluded. Although the study failed to support the hypothesis that depersonalization feeds psychotic delusions, it was based on the unwarranted assumption that feelings of unreality disappear as depersonalization drives the formation of delusions.

It has long been suggested that the presence of depersonalization renders depression resistant to treatment (Mayer-Gross, 1935; Saperstein, 1949). An early controlled study found that study patients with 'neurotic' depression complaining of depersonalization did not benefit from electroconvulsive therapy (ECT) (Ackner, 1960). Similar findings were obtained in a study on 442 patients with depression treated with ETC. It was found that the presence of depersonalization was associated with a poor treatment outcome (Nystrom, 1964). Likewise, it has been reported that depersonalization in the context of depression might constitute a clinical marker of resistance to pharmacotherapy (Nuller, 1982). Along the same lines, it has been found that the absence of depersonalization in depressive patients predicts responsiveness to sleep deprivation therapy (Shelton and Loosen, 1993).

Depersonalization and schizophrenia

Anomalies in the experience of the self have long been thought as being essential components of the clinical picture of schizophrenia. In this regard some writers came to view cases of chronic depersonalization wrongly as mild or subclinical forms of schizophrenia (termed 'pseudoneurotic schizophrenia) (Galdston, 1947; Winnik, 1948). Such assertions were hardly amenable to empirical validation and were based on circular arguments, based on a definition of schizophrenia which emphasized depersonalization-like experiences as core components of the condition. Such a contention still finds resonance in claims that lasting depersonalization is mainly a manifestation of so-called 'schizophrenia spectrum disorders', and which cast doubt on the validity of 'depersonalization disorder' as a chronic condition in its own right (Parnas and Handest, 2003). However, the current view that chronic depersonalization and schizophrenia are unrelated conditions is far from new. For example, in their classic textbook of clinical psychiatry, Mayer-Gross et al. (1969) stated that there was "no evidence that depersonalization sustained for months or years without complicating psychotic features bears any relationship to schizophrenic illness" (p. 122). Current large series of patients with depersonalization disorder clearly support this observation, and show that, as a rule, chronic depersonalization tends to remains stable for decades without giving rise to psychotic conditions (Baker et al., 2003; Simeon et al., 2003b). Furthermore, patients with depersonalization disorder have not been found to be more prone to 'magical thinking' than healthy controls, and scores on dissociation and schizotypy have not been found to correlate (Simeon et al., 2004). It is not clear if patients with schizophrenia are more predisposed to depersonalization experiences. For example, while Spitzer et al. (1997) found that patients with schizophrenia reported more dissociative symptoms than healthy controls another study did not find this to be the case (Brunner *et al.*, 2004). Be that as it may, it would seem that full-blown depersonalization experiences are a rare occurrence in chronic schizophrenia (Sedman, 1963).

The prevalence of depersonalization (at time of study) in patients with schizophrenia has been reported as ranging from 6.9%–11.1% (Hunter *et al.*, 2004), and, as is the case for other psychiatric conditions, its presence seems associated with concomitant anxiety (Noyes *et al.*, 1977). There is, however, some evidence that the presence of depersonalization in patients with schizophrenia affects the clinical presentation and course of the illness itself. One study comparing schizophrenic patients with and without depersonalization found that the former had higher levels of cognitive disturbance, were more sensitive to stress and had greater alexythymia (Maggini *et al.*, 2002). Another study found that schizophrenic patients with depersonalization had more suicidal ideation than those without. Although in this study the presence of akathisia predicted both suicidality and depersonalization, the authors proposed the idea that, rather than being independent constructs, depersonalization and distress may be core subjective components of akathisia itself. In fact, most patients experiencing depersonalization complained of subjective distress regardless of motor manifestations of akathisia (Cem Atbaşoglu *et al.*, 2001).

Some studies have suggested that depersonalization is more frequent in acute schizophrenia than in chronic and disorganized types. Indeed, there is evidence that the presence of derealization constitutes a good prognostic marker in non-disorganized forms of schizophrenia (Varsamis and Adamson, 1971; Hwu *et al.*, 1981).

Depersonalization and pre-psychotic states

Researchers have drawn attention to the occurrence of depersonalization, particularly during the prodromal and acute phase of schizophrenia (Klosterkötter *et al.*, 2008). Indeed, as stated by Mayer-Gross *et al.* (1969): "When depersonalization does occur during the evolution of unquestionable schizophrenic psychosis, it is fleeting in character, the clinical events march swiftly and delusional and hallucinatory experiences are never very far off" (p. 122).

Rather than being specific to schizophrenia, it is more likely that depersonalization constitutes a general feature of pre-psychotic states, regardless of aetiology. For example, one group of researchers found that, in its early stages, the prodrome of schizophrenia was indistinguishable from that of major depression (Häfner *et al.*, 2005). In fact, as was mentioned in relation to depression, several researchers have suggested that, as a psychotic episode evolves, prodromal depersonalization feelings become integrated into emerging delusional systems, a process that has been termed 'psychotic re-personalization'. For example, early writers observed that in the prodromal stage of some psychoses, patients showed smooth transitions from typical depersonalization to a delusional elaboration of the same experiences (Mayer-Gross, 1935; Ackner, 1954; Schilder, 1914). This was interpreted as suggesting that at least some delusions might be based on depersonalization experiences. Thus depersonalization might serve as a general 'experiential substratum' which (modulated by different cognitive frames) will crystallize out into different delusional phenomena (Fuentenebro and Berrios, 1995). In particular, it has been suggested that some forms of nihilistic or hypochondriacal delusions could have their origin in somatic depersonalization experiences, differently conceptualized by the psychotic patient (Cremieux and Cain, 1948; Schilder, 1935; Mayer-Gross, 1935). Attention has also been drawn to the frequent occurrence of depersonalization in patients with Capgras delusions (Christodoulou, 1986), to whose origin 'feelings of unreality' seem causally important. Early writers linked depersonalization to the origin of nihilistic delusions (Ardila and Rosseli, 1988; Basaglia, 1956; Cotard, 1891; Crémieux and Cain, 1948; Séglas, 1889a, b). Recently, a cognitive model has been proposed according to which the phenomenological difference between Capgras and nihilistic delusions would result from paranoid and depressive interpretations, respectively, of underlying depersonalization feelings (Young et al., 1994; Wright, Young and Hellawell, 1993). Similar attributional models have been proposed to explain passivity experiences; for example, "an individual experiencing depersonalization may attribute this experience to witches controlling his or her body, and will thereafter interpret perceptual experiences that are consistent with this belief" (Bryant, 1997).

In terms of differential diagnosis, it is useful to bear in mind that, in addition to depersonalization, pre-psychotic states usually manifest with a range of other phenomena such as thought-related symptoms (interference, blockages, pressure); 'decreased ability to discriminate between ideas and perception, fantasy and true memories'; disturbances of receptive language; unstable ideas of reference; and perception disturbances (Klosterkötter et al., 2008).

Depersonalization as a symptom of dissociative identity disorder (DID) and related chronic dissociative conditions

Depersonalization is a frequent symptom in patients with severe and chronic dissociative conditions whose identity and related autobiographical memory are severely fragmented and compartmentalized into distinct 'ego states' (i.e. 'alters'). A recent study on 220 patients with dissociative identity disorder found the prevalence of depersonalization to be 95% (Dell, 2006), although it tends to episodic rather than constant. A careful assessment of these patients usually reveals a range of symptoms suggestive of severe dissociation such as psychogenic amnesia, time-losing, hallucinatory voices usually experienced within the head, and passivity experiences (Dell, 2006; Putnam, 1989).

Personality disorders and depersonalization

A study of the prevalence of personality disorders amongst 117 patients with depersonalization disorder (Simeon *et al.*, 2003a) found that 52% met diagnostic criteria for at least one of the 14 categories screened (as per DSM-III-R/ DSM-IV, including appendix disorders). While all categories were diagnosed at least once in the sample, three personality disorders stood out as the most frequent: 'avoidant' (23%); 'borderline' (21%); and obsessive-compulsive personality disorder (21%). Interestingly enough, schizotypal and schizoid personality disorder, two categories believed to predispose to schizophrenia, were amongst the least frequently diagnosed in the sample (7% and 4%, respectively).

Avoidant personality disorder

This personality disorder is characterized by pervasive social inhibition and avoidance of social interaction. Patients have deeply rooted feelings of inadequacy, and extreme sensitivity to negative evaluation by others. It is a category which clearly overlaps with social phobia and can be viewed as a particularly severe, persistent and generalized form of social anxiety. In fact, 50%–90% of patients with social phobia are also diagnosed with avoidant personality disorder (Stein and Stein, 2008). Such overlap between the two conditions has cast doubt on the validity of 'avoidant personality disorder' as an independent condition. In this regard, a high prevalence of 'avoidant personality disorder' amongst patients with depersonalization disorder is hardly surprising.

Obsessive-compulsive personality disorder

A high prevalence of obsessional traits such as rigidity, meticulousness and insecurity has been repeatedly observed in patients with chronic and pathological forms of depersonalization (Ziegler, 1929; Grinberg, 1966; Shorvon and Lond, 1947; Roth, 1959; Torch, 1978; Sedman and Reed, 1963). Shorvon (1946), for instance, found obsessional traits in 88% of depersonalization patients. Roth (1959), in turn, reported the presence of premorbid obsessional personalities in 75% of his series. In view of this association, Torch went on to propose the existence of a specific subtype of depersonalization in which obsessional traits seemed to play a causal role: "the syndrome of intellectual-obsessive premorbid personalities is composed of a complex and fascinating combination of alternating states of depersonalization and obsessive self scrutiny" (Torch, 1978, p. 194).

As has been described in other chapters, it has been proposed that depersonalization is triggered by a combined subjective perception of being threatened, coupled with feelings of not being in control. According to such a model, it could be speculated that a personality structure characterized by extreme rigidity and an exaggerated need to be in control, as is the case in individuals with obsessive-compulsive personality disorder, would confer vulnerability to depersonalization by making subjects oversensitive to situations liable to be experienced as threatening and beyond personal control.

Borderline personality disorder

Patients with borderline personality disorder seem also predisposed to experience depersonalization (Hunter, 1966; Benvenuti et al., 2005) as well as other dissociative experiences (Zanarini et al., 2000a). Interestingly, in this particular population, depersonalization would seem to be mainly characterized by intermittent episodes accompanied by intense subjective distress and attempts to bring depersonalization episodes to an end by means of self-harming (Klonsky and Muehlenkamp, 2007; Messer and Fremouw, 2008). "Some who self-injure state that they sometimes feel unreal or feel nothing at all. These experiences can be frightening, and some may use self-injury to interrupt these dissociative episodes. The physical injury or sight of blood may jolt the system and help self-injurers regain a sense of self" (Klonsky and Muehlenkamp, 2007).

At present, the nature of this association is poorly understood, but it would seem to be related to immature defense mechanisms (Wildgoose et al., 2000), a history of sexual trauma and 'something intrinsic' to the borderline personality structure itself (Zanarini et al., 2000b). Ross (2007) compared the prevalence of dissociative symptoms in 93 patients with borderline personality disorder, and 108 without the condition. The main finding was that in-patients with borderline personality disorder reported significantly more dissociative symptoms including depersonalization. Using the Dissociative Disorders Interview Schedule, it was found that 59% of the borderline patients met criteria for a dissociative disorder compared with 22% of the non-borderline patients. This study supports previous findings suggesting that the presence of dissociative symptoms should have added diagnostic weight when ascertaining the presence of borderline personality disorder (Gunderson et al., 1981).

REFERENCES

Ackner, B. (1954). Depersonalisation I. Aetiology and phenomenology. *Journal of Mental Science*, **100**, 838–853.
Ackner, B. (1960). The prognostic significance of depersonalisation in depressive illnesses treated with electroconvulsive therapy. *Journal of Neurology, Neurosurgery and Psychiatry*, **23**, 242–246.

Ali, S. O., Denicoff, K. D., Ketter, T. A., Smith-Jackson, E. E., Post, R. M. (1997). Psychosensory symptoms in bipolar disorder. *Neuropsychiatry, Neuropsychology and Behavioral*, **10**, 223–231.

Ardila, A., Rosseli, M. (1988). Temporal lobe involvement in Capgras syndrome. *International Journal of Neuroscience*, **43**, 219–224.

Baker, D., Hunter, E., Lawrence, E. *et al.* (2003). Depersonalisation disorder: clinical features of 204 cases. *British Journal of Psychiatry*, **182**, 428–433.

Ball, S., Robinson, A., Shekhar, A., Walsh, K. (1997). Dissociative symptoms in panic disorder. *Journal of Nervous and Mental Disease*, **185**, 755–760.

Basaglia, F. (1956). Il corpo nell'hipocondria e nella depersonalizzazione. *Rivista sperimentale di freniatria e medicina Legale delle alienazioni mentali*, **80**, 453–480.

Benedetti, A., Perugi, G., Toni, C., Simonetti, B., Mata, B., Cassano, G. B. (1997). Hypochondriasis and illness phobia in panic–agoraphobic patients. *Comprehensive Psychiatry*, **38**, 124–131.

Benvenuti, A., Rucci, P., Ravani, L. *et al.* (2005). Psychotic features in borderline patients: is there a connection to mood dysregulation? *Bipolar Disorder*, **7**, 338–343.

Bourgeois, M., Jordan, M., Daubech, J. F., Rigal, F., Goumilloux, R., Delile, J. M. (1986). Dépersonnalisation, syndrome de Cotard et virage maniaque sous benzodiazepine (Apropos de deux observations). *Annales Médico-Psychologiques*, **144**, 174–182.

Brauer, R., Harrow, M., Tucker, G. J. (1970). Depersonalization phenomena in psychiatric patients. *British Journal of Psychiatry*, **117**, 509–515.

Breh, D. C., Seidler, G. H. (2007). Is peritraumatic dissociation a risk factor for PTSD? *Journal of Trauma and Dissociation*, **8**, 53–69.

Brunner, R., Parzer, P., Schmitt, R., Resch, F. (2004). Dissociative symptoms in schizophrenia: a comparative analysis of patients with borderline personality disorder and healthy controls. *Psychopathology*, **37**, 281–284.

Bryant, R. (1997). Folie à familie: a cognitive study of delusional beliefs. *Psychiatry*, **60**, 44–50.

Bryant, R. A., Panasetis, P. (2005). The role of panic in acute dissociative reactions following trauma. *British Journal of Clinical Psychology*, **44**, 489–494.

Cardena, E., Spiegel, D. (1993). Dissociative reactions to the San Francisco Bay Area earthquake of 1989. *American Journal of Psychiatry*, **150**, 474–478.

Cassano, G. B., Petracca, A., Perugi, G., Toni, C., Tundo, A., Roth, M. (1989). Derealization and panic attacks: a clinical evaluation on 150 patients with panic disorder/agoraphobia. *Comprehensive Psychiatry*, **30**, 5–12.

Cem Atbaşoglu, E., Schultz, S. K., Andreasen, N. C. (2001). The relationship of akathisia with suicidality and depersonalization among patients with schizophrenia. *The Journal of Neuropsychiatry and Clinical Neuroscience*, **13**, 336–341.

Christodoulou, G. N. (1986). Role of depersonalization-derealization phenomena in the delusional misidentification syndromes. *Bibliotheca Psychiatrica*, **164**, 99–104.

Cotard, J. (1891). Perte de la vision mentale dans la mélancolie anxieuse. *Archives de Neurologie*, **7**, 289–295.

Crémieux, A., Cain, J. (1948). Psychastenie grave avec obsession de négation. *Annales Médico-Psychologiques*, **2**, 76–80.

Dell, P. F. (2006). A new model of dissociative identity disorder. *Psychiatric Clinics of North America*, **29**, 1–26.

Edlund, M., Swann, A., Clothier, J. (1987). Patients with panic attacks and abnormal EEG results. *American Journal of Psychiatry*, **144**, 508–509.

Federn, P. (1926). Some variations in ego feelings. *International Journal of Psychoanalysis*, **2**, 434–444.

Feigenbaum, D. (1937). Depersonalization as defense mechanism. *Psychoanalytic Quarterly*, **6**, 4–11.

Fuentenebro, F., Berrios, G. E. (1995). The predelusional state: a conceptual history. *Comprehensive Psychiatry*, **36**, 251–259.

Galdston, I. (1947). On the aetiology of depersonalisation. *Journal of Nervous and Mental Disease*, **105**, 25–39.

Gittleson, N. L. (1967). A phenomenological test of a theory of depersonalization. *British Journal of Psychiatry*, **113**, 677–678.

Griffin, G. M., Resick, P., Mechanic, M. B. (1997). Objective assessment of peritraumatic dissociation: psychophysiological indicators. *American Journal of Psychiatry*, **154**, 1081–1088.

Grinberg, L. (1966). The relationship between obsessive mechanism and a state of self disturbance: depersonalization. *International Journal of Psychoanalysis*, **46**, 177–183.

Gunderson, J. G., Kolb, J. E., Austin, V. (1981). The diagnostic interview for borderline patients. *American Journal of Psychiatry*, **138**, 896–903.

Häfner, H., Maurer, K., Trendler, G., an der Heiden, W., Schmidt, M., Könnecke, R. (2005). Schizophrenia and depression: challenging the paradigm of two separate diseases – a controlled study of schizophrenia, depression and healthy controls. *Schizophrenia Research*, **77**, 11–24.

Hillman, R. G. (1981). The psychopathology of being held hostage. *American Journal of Psychiatry*, **138**, 1193–1197.

Hollander, E., Fairbanks, J., Decaria, C., Liebowitz, M. R. (1989). Pharmacological dissection of panic and depersonalization. *American Journal of Psychiatry*, **146**, 402.

Hunter, R. C. (1966). The analysis of episodes of depersonalization in a borderline patient. *International Journal of Psychoanalysis*, **47**, 32–41.

Hunter, E. C., Sierra, M., David, A. S. (2004). The epidemiology of depersonalisation and derealisation. A systematic review. *Social Psychiatry and Psychiatric Epidemiology*, **39**, 9–18.

Hwu, H., Chen, C., Tsuang, M., Tseng, W. (1981). Derealization syndrome and the outcome of schizophrenia: a report from the international pilot study of schizophrenia. *British Journal of Psychiatry*, **39**, 313–318.

Juliusburger (1912). Zur Lehre von den Fremdheitsgefühlen. *Monatsschrift für Neurologie und Psychiatrie*, **22**, 270.

Katerndahl, D. A., Talamantes, M. (2000). A comparison of persons with early-versus late-onset panic attacks. *Journal of Clinical Psychiatry*, **61**, 422–427.

Klonsky, E. D., Muehlenkamp, J. J. (2007). Self-injury: a research review for the practitioner. *Journal of Clinical Psychiatry*, **63**, 1045–1056.

Klosterkötter, J., Hellmich, M., Steinmeyer, E. M., Schultze-Lutter, F. (2001). Diagnosing schizophrenia in the initial prodromal phase. *Archives of General Psychiatry*, **58**, 158–164.

Klosterkötter, J., Schultze-Lutter, F., Ruhrmann, S. (2008). Kraepelin and psychotic prodromal conditions. *European Archives of Psychiatry and Clinical Neuroscience*, **258** Suppl, 2, 74–84.

Kraepelin, E. (1896). *Lehrbuch der Psychiatrie*. (5th edition). Leipzig.

Krishaber, M. (1873). *De la Névropathie Cérébro-Cardiaque*. Paris:Masson.

Lachlan, A., McWiliams, M. A., Brian, J., Cox, P. H. D., Murray, W. (2001). Trauma and depersonalization during panic attacks. *American Journal of Psychiatry*, **158**, 656.

Lewis, A. J. (1934). Melancholia: clinical survey of depressive states. *Journal of Mental Science*, **80**, 277–378.

Liebowitz, M..R, McGrath, P. J., Bush, S. C. (1980). Mania occurring during treatment for depersonalization: a report of two cases. *Journal of Clinical Psychiatry*, **41**, 33–34.

Locatelli, M., Bellodi, L., Perna, G., Scarone, S. (1993). EEG power modifications in panic disorder during a temporolimbic activation task: relationships with temporal lobe clinical symptomatology. *The Journal of Neuropsychiatry and Clinical Neurosciences*, **5**, 409–414.

Locatelli, M., Bellodi, L., Perna, G., Scarone, S. (1995). Temporal lobe involvement in panic disorder: results of a replication study. *Journal of Neuropsychiatry*, **7**, 272–273.

Maggini, C., Raballo, A., Salvatore, P. (2002). Depersonalization and basic symptoms in schizophrenia. *Psychopathology*, **35**, 17–24.

Marmar, C. R., Weiss, D. S., Schlenger, W. E. *et al.* (1994). Peritraumatic dissociation and posttraumatic stress in male Vietnam theater veterans. *American Journal of Psychiatry*, **151**, 902–907.

Marshall, R. D., Schneier, F. R., Lin, S. H., Simpson, H. B., Vermes, D., Liebowitz, M. (2000). Childhood trauma and dissociative symptoms in panic disorder. *American Journal of Psychiatry*, **157**, 451–453.

Mayer-Gross, W. (1935). On depersonalisation. *British Journal of Medical Psychology*, **15**, 103–122.

Mayer-Gross, W., Slater, E., Roth, M. (1969). *Clinical Psychiatry*, 3rd edn. London: Martin. Baillière, Tindall & Cassell.

Medford, N., Baker, D., Hunter, E. *et al.* (2003). Chronic depersonalization following illicit drug use: a controlled analysis of 40 cases. *Addiction*, **98**, 1731–1736.

Messer, J. M., Fremouw, W. J. (2008). A critical review of explanatory models for self-mutilating behaviors in adolescents. *Clinical Psychology Reviews*, **28**, 162–178.

Michal, M., Sann, U., Grabhorn, R., Overbeck, G., Röder, Ch. (2005b). Zur Prävalenz von Depersonalisation und Derealisation in der stationären Psychotherapie. *Psychotherapeut*, **50**, 328–339.

Michal, M., Kaufhold, J., Grabhorn, R., Krakow, K., Overbeck, G., Heidenreich, T. (2005a). Depersonalization and social anxiety. *Journal of Nervous and Mental Disease*, **193**, 629–632.

Michal, M., Heidenreich, T., Engelbach, U. *et al.* (2006). Depersonalisation, soziale Ängste und Scham. *Psychotherapie, Psychosomatik, Medizinische Psychologie*, **56**, 383–389.

Michal, M., Beutel, M. E., Jordan, J., Zimmermann, M., Wolters, S., Heidenreich, T. (2007). Depersonalization, mindfulness, and childhood trauma. *Journal of Nervous and Mental Disease*, **195**, 693–696.

Mula, M., Pini, S., Cassano, G. B. (2007). The neurobiology and clinical significance of depersonalization in mood and anxiety disorders: a critical reappraisal. *Journal of Affective Disorders*, **99**, 91–99.

Mula, M., Pini, S., Preve, M., Masini, M., Giovannini, I., Cassano, E. B. (2008). Clinical correlates of depersonalization symptoms in patients with bipolar disorder. *Journal of Affective Disorders*, Sept 9. [Epub ahead of Print].

Nixon, R. D., Resick, P. A., Griffin, M. G. (2004). Panic following trauma: the etiology of acute posttraumatic arousal. *Journal of Anxiety Disorder*, **18**, 193–210.

Noyes, R., Kletti, R. (1977). Depersonalisation in response to life threatening danger. *Comprehensive Psychiatry*, **18**, 375–384.

Noyes, R., Hoenk, P. R., Kuperman, S., Slymen, D. J. (1977). Depersonalization in accident victims and psychiatric patients. *Journal of Nervous and Mental Disease*, **164**, 401–407.

Noyes, R. Jr., Woodman, C., Garvey, M. J. *et al.* (1992). Generalized anxiety disorder vs. panic disorder. Distinguishing characteristics and patterns of comorbidity. *Journal of Nervous and Mental Disease*, **180**, 369–379.

Nuller, Y. L. (1982). Depersonalisation: symptoms, meaning, therapy. *Acta Psychiatrica Scandinavica*, **66**, 451–458.

Nystrom, S. (1964). On the relation between clinical factors and efficacy of ECT in depression. *Acta Psychiatrica Scandinavica*, Suppl, **181**, 1–140.

Oberndorf, C. P. (1935). Genesis of feeling of unreality (depersonalization). *International Journal of Psychoanalysis*, **16**, 296–306.

Oberndorf, C.P (1950). The role of anxiety in depersonalisation. *International Journal of Psychoanalysis*, **31**, 1–5.

Parnas, J., Handest, P. (2003). Phenomenology of anomalous self-experience in early schizophrenia. *Comprehensive Psychiatry*, **44**, 121–134.

Phillips, M..L, Sierra, M. (2003). Depersonalization disorder: a functional neuroanatomical perspective. *Stress*, **6**, 157–165.

Putnam, F. W. (1989). *Diagnosis and Treatment of Multiple Personality Disorder*. New York: The Guilford Press.

Ross, C. A. (2007). Borderline personality disorder and dissociation. *Journal of Trauma and Dissociation*, **8**, 71–80.

Roth, M. (1959). The phobic anxiety-depersonalisation syndrome. *Proceedings of the Royal Society of Medicine*, **52**, 587–595.

Saperstein, J. L. (1949). Phenomena of depersonalization. *Journal of Nervous and Mental Disease*, **110**, 236–251.

Schilder, P. (1938). The social neurosis. *Psychoanalitic Review*, **25**, 1–19.

Schilder, P. (1914). *Selbstbewusstsein und Persönlichkeitbewusstsein: eine psychopathologische Studie*. Berlin:Verlag von Julius Springer.

Schilder, P. (1935). *The Image and Appearance of the Human Body*. London: Kegan Paul.

Schönenberg, M., Reichwald, U., Domes, G., Badke, A., Hautzinger, M. (2005). Effects of peritraumatic ketamine medication on early and sustained posttraumatic stress symptoms in moderately injured accident victims. *Psychopharmacology (Berlin)*, **182**, 420–425.

Schönenberg, M., Reichwald, V., Domes, G., Badke, A., Hautzinger, M. (2008). Ketamine aggravates symptoms of acute stress disorder in a naturalistic sample of accident victims. *Journal of Psychopharmacology*, **22**, 493–497.

Sedman, G. (1963). Depersonalization and mood changes in schizophrenia. *British Journal of Psychiatry*, **109**, 669–673.

Sedman, G., Reed, G. F. (1963). Depersonalization phenomena in obsessional personalities and in depression. *British Journal of Psychiatry*, **109**, 376–379.

Seemüller, F., Riedel, M., Wickelmaier, F. *et al.* (2008). Atypical symptoms in hospitalised patients with major depressive episode: frequency, clinical characteristics, and internal validity. *Journal of Affective Disorders*, **108**, 271–278.

Séglas, J. (1889a). Semiologie et pathogénie des idées de négation (Les alterations de la personalité dans les délires melancoliques). *Annales Médico-Psychologiques*, **47**, 5–26.

Séglas, J. (1889b). Les alterations de la personalité dans le délire de négation. *Annales Médico-Psychologiques*, **10**, 5.

Segui, J., Marquez, M., Garcia, L., Canet, J., Salvador-Carulla, L., Ortiz, M. (2000). Depersonalization in panic disorder: a clinical study. *Psychiatry*, **41**, 172–178.

Shäfer, (no initial) (1880). Bemerkungen zur psychiatrischen Formenlehre. *Allgemeine Zeitschrift für Psychiatrie*, **36**, 214–278.

Shelton, R., Loosen, P. (1993). Sleep deprivation accelerates the response to nortriptyline. *Progress in Neuropsychopharmacology and Biological Psychiatry*, **17**, 113–123.

Shilony, E., Grossman, F. (1993). Depersonalization as a defense mechanism in survivors of trauma. *Journal of Traumatic Stress*, **6**, 119–128.

Shorvon, H. J. (1946). The depersonalisation syndrome. *Proceedings of the Royal Society of Medicine*, **39**, 779–792.

Shorvon, H. J., Lond, M. B. (1947). Prefrontal leucotomy and the depersonalisation syndrome. *The Lancet*, **2**, 714–718.

Sierra, M., Berrios, G. E. (1998). Depersonalization: neurobiological perspectives. *Biological Psychiatry*, **44**, 898–908.

Sierra, M. (2008). Depersonalization disorder: pharmacological approaches. *Expert Review of Neurotherapeutics*, **8**, 19–26.

Sierra, M., Berrios, G. E. (2000). The Cambridge Depersonalization Scale: a new instrument for the measurement of depersonalization. *Psychiatry Research*, **93**, 153–164.

Silberman, E. K., Post, R. M., Nurnberger, J., Theodore, W., Boulenger, J. P. (1985). Transient sensory, cognitive and affective phenomena in affective illness: a comparison with complex partial epilepsy. *British Journal of Psychiatry*, **146**, 81–89.

Simeon, D., Guralnik, O., Schmeidler, J., Sirof, B., Knutelska, M. (2001). The role of childhood interpersonal trauma in depersonalization disorder. *American Journal of Psychiatry*, **158**, 1027–1033.

Simeon, D., Knutelska, M., Nelson, D., Guralnik, O. (2003a). Feeling unreal: a depersonalization disorder update of 117 cases. *Journal of Clinical Psychiatry*, **64**, 990–997.

Simeon, D., Riggio-Rosen, A., Guralnik, O., Knutelska, M., Nelson, D. (2003b). Depersonalization disorder: dissociation and affect. *Journal of Trauma and Dissociation*, **4**, 63–76.

Simeon, D., Guralnik, O., Knutelska, M., Nelson, D. (2004). Dissection of schizotypy and dissociation in depersonalization disorder. *Journal of Trauma and Dissociation*, **5**, 111–119.

Sloan, P. (1988). Post-traumatic stress in survivors of an airplane crash-landing: A clinical and exploratory research intervention. *Journal of Traumatic Stress*, **1**, 211–229.

Spiegel, D., Classen, C., Cardena, E. (2000). New DSM-IV diagnosis of acute stress disorder. *American Journal of Psychiatry*, **157**, 1890–1891.

Spitzer, C., Haug, H. J., Freyberger, H. J. (1997). Dissociative symptoms in schizophrenic patients with positive and negative symptoms. *Psychopathology*, **30**, 67–75.

Stein, M. B., Stein, D. J. (2008). Social anxiety disorder. *Lancet*, **371**, 1115–1125.

Steinberg, M. (1991). The spectrum of depersonalization: assessment and treatment. In Tasman, A., Goldfinger, S. M. (eds), *APA Review of Psychiatry*, **10**, 223–247.

Steinberg, M., Rounsaville, B., Cicchetti, D. V. (1990). The Structured Clinical Interview for DSM-III-R Dissociative Disorders: preliminary report on a new diagnostic instrument. *American Journal of Psychiatry*, **147**, 76–82.

Swinson, R. P., Kuch, K. (1990). Clinical features of panic and related disorders. In Ballenger, J. C. (ed.), *Clinical Aspects of Panic Disorder. Frontiers of Clinical Neuroscience* (Vol. 9). New York, NY: Wiley-Liss, pp. 13–30.

Taal, L. A., Faber, A. W. (1997). Dissociation as a predictor of psychopathology following burns injury. *Burns*, **23**, 400–403.

Torch, E. M. (1978). Review of the relationship between obsession and depersonalisation. *Acta Psychiatrica Scandinavica*, **58**, 191–198.

Trueman, D. (1984). Anxiety and depersonalization and derealization experiences. *Psychological Reports*, **54**, 91–96.

Varsamis, J., Adamson, J. D. (1971). Early schizophrenia. *Canadian Psychiatric Association Journal*, **6**, 487–497.

Wildgoose, A., Waller, G., Clarke, S., Reid, A. (2000). Psychiatric symptomatology in borderline and other personality disorders: dissociation and fragmentation as mediators. *Journal of Nervous and Mental Disease*, **188**, 757–763.

Wilkinson, C. B. (1983). Aftermath of a disaster: the collapse of the Hyatt Regency Hotel skywalks. *American Journal of Psychiatry*, **140**, 1134–1139.

Winnik, H. (1947–1948). On the structure of the depersonalization neurosis. *British Journal of Medical Psychology*, **21**, 268–277.

World Health Organization (1992). F48.1. Depersonalisation-derealisation syndrome. In *The ICD-10 Classification of Mental and Behavioural Disorders. Clinical Descriptions and Diagnostic Guidelines*. Geneva: World Health Organization, pp. 171–173.

Wright, S., Young, A. W., Hellawell, D. J. (1993). Sequential Cotard and Capgras delusions. *British Journal of Clinical Psychology*, **32**, 345–349.

Young, A. W., Leafhead, K. M., Szulecka, T. K. (1994). The Capgras and Cotard delusions. *Psychopathology*, **27**, 226–231.

Zanarini, M. C., Ruser, T., Frankenburg, F. R., Hennen, J. (2000a). The dissociative experiences of borderline patients. *Comprehensive Psychiatry*, **41**, 223–227.

Zanarini, M. C., Ruser, T. F., Frankenburg, F. R., Hennen, J., Gunderson, J. G. (2000b). Risk factors associated with the dissociative experiences of borderline patients. *Journal of Nervous and Mental Disease*, **188**, 26–30.

Ziegler, L. H. (1929). Compulsions, obsessions and feelings of unreality. *Human Biology*, **1**, 514–527.

Zoellner, L. A., Jaycox, L. H., Watlington, C. G., Foa, E. B. (2003). Are the dissociative criteria in ASD useful? *Journal of Trauma and Stress*, **16**, 341–350.

6

Depersonalization in neurology

Introduction

It has long been observed that depersonalization can occur in patients with a wide range of neurological and psychiatric conditions. It was indeed this apparent lack of specificity that led some researchers to view depersonalization as a kind of predetermined brain response not unlike stereotyped manifestations of a neurological insult such as delirium or seizures (Mayer-Gross, 1935). As early as 1936, the German neuropsychiatrist K. Haug wrote an entire monograph in which he reported in exquisite detail series of cases with a variety of neurological pathology such as head injuries, strokes, encephalitis, intoxications, etc., all of which manifested severe depersonalization as the most prominent symptom (Haug, 1936). Subsequent anecdotal reports have confirmed these associations (Frank, 1934; Brock and Wiesel, 1942; Heuyer and Serin, 1920; Heuyer and Dublineau, 1932) and have added new ones such as Menière's Disease (Grigsby, 1986), multiple sclerosis (Ströhle *et al.*, 2000), and acute intermittent porphyria (Lambert *et al.*, 2003). A systematic review of all published cases found epilepsy and migraine to be the most commonly associated neurological diagnoses (Lambert *et al.*, 2003). This chapter will deal with only those neurological conditions whose association with depersonalization has been researched systematically. These conditions are: epilepsy, migraine, head injury, inner ear disease and sleep disorders.

Depersonalization and epilepsy

The relationship between depersonalization and epilepsy has been more systematic and more reliably reported than any other neuropsychiatric condition. As early as 1869, Griesinger (1868–69) described experiences redolent of depersonalization (the term had not been coined yet) as part of the epileptic syndrome: "Some [epileptic] patients declare themselves quite unable to describe the type of sensory anomalies they experience. One said: "perceptions emerge into consciousness in a way that cannot be defined but only described by saying that they seem as if they were different. The singing of birds sounds different to me, as do the utterances of my relatives; the air feels different, and the body feels as if made from another material…;" (p. 328). Hughlings Jackson (1889) reported similar depersonalization-like experiences as part of what he termed 'epileptic dreamy states'. Pick (1909), in turn, suggested a related mechanism between depersonalization and epileptic seizures: "Although I am not prepared to conclude that the symptomatology of my [depersonalized] patient is *entirely* to be understood as a form of epilepsy, I believe that the psychological similarity is too significant to refrain from likening their clinical pictures" (Pick 1903; Translated by Viviani and Berrios 1996; p. 331). Roth and Harper (1962) also found a phenomenological similarity between depersonalization states and temporal lobe epilepsy, and believed that the fact that both states could be accompanied by panic attacks and agoraphobia suggested the presence of a temporal lobe mechanism in depersonalization. Based on their finding that only patients with anxiety neurosis (so-called phobic–anxiety–depersonalization syndrome) reported derealization, these researchers also suggested that this symptom could discriminate between TLE and anxiety neurosis. This has not been confirmed by later studies; for example, one study found that patients with 'affective disorders' and TLE showed a similar frequency of depersonalization and derealization (Silberman *et al.*, 1985). Likewise, other authors have reported that, out of 128 patients with complex partial seizures, 18% experienced ictal derealization and 15% ictal depersonalization; the same experiences occurred interictally in 14% and 10% of cases, respectively (Devinsky *et al.*, 1991).

In yet another interesting study, researchers found features of depersonalization and derealization in 61% of a sample of 41 patients with complex partial seizures (Toni *et al.*, 1996), although they did not specify the timing of the experiences with regard to the occurrence of seizures. Another study exploring the relationship between epilepsy and dissociative predisposition (Devinsky *et al.*, 1989) compared dissociation scores (as measured by the Dissociative Experiences Scale) between 71 patients with epilepsy (12 with generalized and 59 with complex partial seizures); 42 patients with multiple personality disorder, a chronic and severe dissociative condition (now called dissociative identity disorder by DSM-IV); and 34 normal controls. The main finding was that patients with epilepsy had higher dissociation scores than normal controls, but lower than those of patients with dissociative disorder. In fact, within the epileptic group, those suffering from partial seizures had higher dissociation scores than those affected by generalized seizures. Furthermore, patients with dominant hemisphere foci scored higher on a subscale specific to depersonalization than those with non-dominant foci. In the same vein, another study compared a group of patients with complex partial epilepsy, with groups of

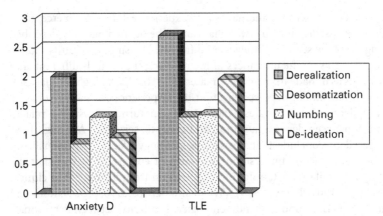

Fig. 6.1. Comparison of depersonalization symptoms between patients with anxiety disorders and patients with temporal lobe epilepsy (TLE). The latter group had significantly higher CDS scores on the desomatization and the de-ideation scale (P < 0.05).

patients suffering from post-traumatic stress disorders and anxiety disorders, and a group of normal controls (Persinger and Makarec, 1993). It was found that the epileptic patients obtained the highest depersonalization scores across all groups. Another study compared the phenomenology of depersonalization symptoms of patients with depersonalization disorder with a group of patients with temporal lobe epilepsy, and another one with anxiety disorders. Whilst depersonalization disorder was found to be characterized by long-lasting, intense depersonalization experiences, both the anxiety and the epilepsy groups experienced fleeting episodes of depersonalization, usually lasting from a few seconds to a few minutes (Sierra and Berrios, 2000). A comparison of the latter two groups along the symptom domains of depersonalization (see Fig. 6.1), revealed that patients with temporal lobe epilepsy report significantly more 'anomalous body experiences' as well as more memory-related complaints ('subjective anomalies of recall'). It would seem to be the case that the occurrence of depersonalization-like symptoms in epileptic patients is somewhat specific to temporal lobe seizures. However, in contrast to the above findings, a recent study used measures of depersonalization and dissociation (Cambridge Depersonalization Scale and Dissociative Experiences Scale, respectively) to compare 37 patients with a diagnosis of epilepsy regardless of seizure type or focus and 32 patients with non-epileptic seizures (Lawton *et al.*, 2008). Interestingly, both groups scored well below diagnostic cut-off points on both scales, with no significant differences between the two groups.

From what has been reviewed so far, it would seem that the presence of episodic depersonalization, particularly when accompanied by prominent and paroxysmal distortions in body experiencing, and in the experience of time, should raise suspicion to the possibility of temporal lobe epilepsy, particularly if the episodes are attended by consciousness clouding, and are accompanied by other 'psychosensory' symptoms such as déjà vu, forced thinking, etc. (Devinsky and Luciano, 1991). However, establishing an epileptic source for episodic depersonalization experiences is not an easy endeavour, even in already diagnosed epileptic patients (Kanemoto, 1997). A case recently discussed illustrates well such a diagnostic conundrum (Dietl *et al.*, 2005). The patient was a 39-year-old woman who, in addition to experiencing well-documented 'grand mal' epileptic seizures complained of intermittent 'altered states of consciousness' lasting several days, during which she felt "strangely altered" and "unreal." She experienced her environment as 'far away' or 'covered by an invisible veil.' During such states she felt her body 'weightless, like floating in the air'. Sometimes she felt completely 'out of her body'. She felt like having 'the thoughts and movements of a robot' (Dietl *et al.*, 2005). Particularly suggestive of an epileptic aetiology was the fact that, during these depersonalization episodes, she also experienced 'strange tastes and smells (e.g. like the smell of a cigarette) and nausea'. An interictal positron emission tomography scan revealed right-sided temporomesial hypometabolism. During depersonalization episodes, however, a focal area of hyperperfusion was observed in the right amygdala. Long-term continuous EEG also recorded right-sided temporal sharp waves. However, in spite of all this supporting evidence, it was impossible to ascertain an epileptic origin, given that long-term video/EEG revealed no evidence of seizure activity during depersonalization episodes, and the patient did not improve with anticonvulsant trials.

Although there have been studies suggesting a relationship between intermittent depersonalization episodes and electroencephalographic anomalies in the temporal lobes (Locatelli *et al.*, 1993), EEG screening of patients suffering with constant depersonalization (i.e. depersonalization disorder) have not been revealing (Shorvon, 1946; Davidson, 1964).

Depersonalization and migraine

Shorvon (1946) was the first to report an association between depersonalization and migraine headaches. In his series of 66 patients with pathological depersonalization, he found that 38% had a history of migraine. A similar observation was made by others at the time (Todd, 1963; Davidson, 1964). In the series of 204 patients with depersonalization disorder, it was found that 31% had a self-reported history of headaches (a diagnosis of migraine was not established) and, of these, one-third believed that their headaches and depersonalization were connected (Baker *et al.*, 2003). However, in the other large series of patients, it was found that only 13% of 117 cases had a history of migraine (Simeon *et al.*, 2003).

The precise nature of the association between migraine and depersonalization is currently unknown. Such symptoms may occur as a component of migraine auras (Sacks, 1992), or may happen in the interval between termination or aura and the onset of headache (see below). Somesthesic migraine auras characterized by dramatic distortions in body experience, such as magnification of body parts, can be accompanied by depersonalization (Kew *et al.*, 1998; Podoll and Ebel, 1998). A dramatic example of this is the so-called Alice in Wonderland syndrome. The latter is most commonly reported in children, and is characterized by the occurrence of a somesthesic aura often accompanied by depersonalization, visual illusions and distortions in the perception of time (Todd, 1963). Certain types of migraine such as basilar migraine seem particularly predisposing to altered states of consciousness, to the point that the latter may at times eclipse other more common clinical features: "one must consider the possible diagnosis of atypical migraine when paroxysmal and periodic shifts of mental states are seen in a child or adolescent with a positive familial history of migraine" (Pelletier *et al.*, 1995).

In addition to its occurrence as a migraine aura, depersonalization has also been known to occur during the interval between the termination of aura and the onset of headache. Such a period of time can last from a few minutes to a few hours and is known as the 'free interval'. A study providing detailed clinical descriptions on the 'free interval' of 25 migraine patients experiencing visual auras found that 88% of them experienced symptoms suggestive of depersonalization: "Most had difficulties describing them [the symptoms], using expressions such as 'very strange', 'unreal', 'removed from surroundings'; 'away from everything'; 'not with it'; 'spread out – as though a barrier between me and others'; 'curious feelings of unreality'" (Blau, 1992). One of the patients intimated that "she had never told anyone about the sensations during this phase of migraines, because she felt herself to be insane during these intervals that in her case lasted 20–30 minutes" (Blau, 1992).

In migraineurs depersonalization can also occur as a premonitory symptom preceding a migraine attack, or can happen as a residual state following the headache episode: "My migraine experience starts with hunger. I suddenly feel hungry. Shortly after that my vision becomes 'distant'. It is somewhat like seeing the world projected on a screen. The actual experience is not that obviously artificial, but that is the closest that I can come to conveying the feeling" (Podoll, 2005).

Shorvon (1946) made the puzzling observation that, frequently, the onset of depersonalization in a migraine sufferer seemed to coincide with a cessation or decreased frequency of headache episodes. Some cases seen by the author seem to bear out that observation:

A 35-year-old male with a 5-year history of constant depersonalization (depersonalization disorder), reported a life-time history of frequent migraine attacks whose onset would be preceded by transient depersonalization-like feelings. He had noted, however, that following the onset of constant depersonalization, his migraine attacks ceased to occur. In fact, he described his constant depersonalization as a feeling "that I'm about to have a migraine attack, but it never comes".

It has been suggested that some cases of depersonalization disorder could represent undiagnosed cases of migraine with prolonged aura (Cahill and Murphy, 2004) (one or more aura symptoms lasting >60 min and ≤ 7 days), or even aura status without headache (Kunkel, 2005). According to this suggestion, depersonalization/derealization occurring in the context of migrainous aura could uncommonly follow a protracted course. Persisting migraine aura symptoms are rare but well documented and most commonly take the form of visual perseverations such as 'visual snow', 'TV static' or after-images. These symptoms are often bilateral and may last for weeks, months or years. Intriguingly enough, some patients with depersonalization disorder report a range of visual symptoms such as 'flashes of light', or 'visual snow' which are indeed redolent of migraine auras. In our series of patients (Baker *et al.*, 2003) 41.3% reported flashes of light, which ranged from infrequent to all the time. In fact, patients with a history of recurrent headaches had higher frequencies of flashes of light and other symptoms such as tinnitus than patients without a history of headaches. In view of the above findings, it has been proposed that a proportion of cases diagnosed with depersonalization disorder could in fact be suffering from protracted migraine aura status (Cahill and Murphy, 2004). This possibility is unlikely. A significant proportion of patients with depersonalization disorder experience the condition continuously for more than a decade, which would be exceptionally rare for persistent aura states. Additionally, the condition has been associated with a number of clinical and neurobiological findings not commonly found in migraine patients (Baker *et al.*, 2003; Phillips and Sierra, 2003). Nevertheless, the possibility of identifying a subgroup of patients in whom migraine plays a relevant role in symptomatology and course of illness, is certainly a topic which merits further research.

Depersonalization following head trauma

The occurrence of depersonalization in the aftermath of head injury is a fairly well-documented albeit poorly understood observation. This is in part due to the fact that most reports have been limited to single or very few cases (Grigsby, 1986; Chong, 1995; Paulig *et al.*, 1998). A notable exception however, is a study by Grigsby and Kaye (1993), in which 70 head-trauma patients were rigorously assessed to determine the incidence of depersonalization by means of the Structured Clinical Interview for DSM-III-R Dissociative Disorders (SCID-D). Rather surprisingly, it was found that 50% of cases had experienced depersonalization following the injury. In 66% of those affected, the onset of depersonalization was immediate, while in 20% the onset was delayed by 1–14 days. Rather than being a fleeting occurrence, it was found that, in nearly half the patients, depersonalization had remained constant since its onset or was characterized by frequently recurring episodes. In both clinical presentations patients remained symptomatic for at least 3 months. In fact, only 6% of those affected by depersonalization experienced it as a temporary isolated occurrence at the time of injury. As is usually the case with depersonalization disorder, most affected patients experienced depersonalization as an extremely distressing condition and a substantial group reported fears of going mad.

Interestingly enough, the authors found a significant negative correlation ($r = -0.40$) between the length of time patients remained unconscious following the trauma and the subsequent occurrence of depersonalization (Grigsby and Kaye, 1993). Thus, while 67% of those patients who did not lose consciousness or lost it for less than 30 minutes, experienced depersonalization, only 11% of those with longer times of unconsciousness went on to experience the condition.

Neuropsychological testing failed to reveal any association between cognitive impairment and depersonalization. Likewise, personality tests failed to reveal any personality types as predisposing to experience the condition.

The mechanisms responsible for the occurrence of depersonalization after head trauma remain poorly understood. Although it has been suggested that frontal and temporal lesions play a facilitating role in patients with severe trauma (Paulig et al., 1998), it is unlikely that localized lesions are of relevance among most patients with minor head trauma. In this regard, it has been proposed that depersonalization could be a manifestation of 'subtle', non-localized brain damage leading to 'problems with the integration of perceptual, affective and attentional information' (Grigsby and Kaye, 1993). An alternative hypothesis, however, could be that depersonalization is mediated by a psychological reaction to the traumatic event rather than being 'organically' determined. In support of this, it has been found that as many as 51% of those patients complaining of depersonalization also met DSM-III-R criteria for post-traumatic stress disorder (PTSD) (Grigsby and Kaye, 1993). This finding is interesting in view of studies which have shown that the presence of depersonalization-like experiences in the wake of a traumatic event (i.e. 'peritraumatic dissociation'), predicts the subsequent occurrence of PTSD (see Chapter 4).

A more physiologically based hypothesis posits that depersonalization is related to vestibular symptoms which frequently occur following minor head trauma, such as vertigo, dizziness or light-headedness (Hoffer et al., 2007). Indeed, as will be seen in the next section, there is evidence suggesting that vestibular dysfunction can frequently trigger depersonalization symptoms. Supporting this view, it was found that, in the ten patients who developed vertigo, 80% reported depersonalization. The fact remains, however, that vertigo and depersonalization did not coexist in the majority of cases (Grigsby and Kaye, 1993). It is clear that the occurrence of depersonalization after head trauma is a common and poorly understood phenomenon, which in all likelihood involves a convergence of psychological as well as neurobiological mechanisms. Unfortunately, the scarcity of publications and research in this area is bound to be reflecting a similar neglect in clinical practice. This is a most unfortunate situation, given the high levels of distress that normally accompany depersonalization. Unlike the case with non-specific cognitive symptoms of the 'post-concussional syndrome', such as memory and concentration difficulties, depersonalization is an ineffable, anxiety-provoking state of mind, perceived as discontinuous with 'ordinary consciousness'. It is hardly surprising that undiagnosed patients often bear in silence a tremendous fear of going mad. The importance of identifying and diagnosing depersonalization in head trauma patients cannot be overemphasized, given that its detection and psycho-education alone can be enough to help alleviate anxiety levels significantly (Grigsby, 1986; Hunter *et al.*, 2003).

Depersonalization and vestibular disease

An association between depersonalization and vestibular symptoms such as vertigo or 'lightheadedness' has long been observed. In fact, most of the patients originally described by Krishaber as suffering from 'unreality feelings' (the term depersonalization had not yet been coined) also suffered from severe and incapacitating vertigo (Krishaber, 1873). It was, however, the great German neuropsychiatrist Paul Schilder (1935) who first elaborated in depth on this association: "I first pointed out that there are very close relationships between the vestibular apparatus and depersonalization, and since then I have always emphasised this connection" (p. 167). Although Schilder was adamant on the psychogenic origin of depersonalization, he conceded that "dizziness due to organic causes often provokes phenomena which are akin to the psychic phenomena of depersonalization of the body" (p. 140).

According to Schilder, in view of the central role played by the vestibular apparatus on the integration of body image, any psychological disruption in the latter would manifest itself as if an organic vestibular lesion had taken place. As a corollary, however, physiological dysfunction in the vestibular apparatus would be expected to give rise to depersonalization feelings as a consequence of its effects on body representation. It has indeed been reported that vestibular disease can cause depersonalization (Grigsby and Johnston, 1989). In fact, Sang *et al.* (2006) carried out a systematic study looking at the prevalence of depersonalization in 50 patients with vestibular dysfunction as compared with 121 healthy controls. Using a 28-item self-rating scale (Cox and Swinson, 2002), it was found that all the vestibular patients obtained significantly higher depersonalization scores than the controls. Furthermore, the fact that most patients endorsed a whole range of items pertaining to the different symptom domains of depersonalization (see Fig. 6.2), suggests that they were indeed experiencing a full-fledged depersonalization syndrome, rather than just re-describing an experience of vertigo and dizziness by means of suitable scale items. This notwithstanding, it

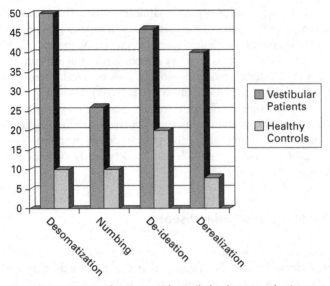

Fig. 6.2. Percentage of patients with vestibular disease endorsing representative items of four symptom domains: (1) desomatization: 'body feels strange or different in some way'; (2) numbing: 'numbing of emotions'; (3) de-ideation:'thoughts seem blurred'; (4) derealization: 'surroundings seem strange and unreal'. (Adapted from Sang et al., 2006.)

is interesting that the prevalence of emotional numbing seemed far lower to that reported in patients with depersonalization disorder.

In a second phase of the study, the researchers were able to induce depersonalization experimentally in 20 normal controls by means of a caloric stimulation test. It would seem that a sensory mismatch between disordered vestibular input and other sensory signals impairs the process whereby an ongoing representation of the body within the surrounding space is achieved (Jáuregui-Renaud et al., 2008). More specifically, it has been proposed that vestibular and multisensory information becomes integrated in a cortical region known as the temporoparietal junction (Lenggenhager et al., 2006). This area has been shown to be relevant in the generation of the experience of being localized within one's body (i.e. embodiment).

Depersonalization and sleep disorders

Patients with depersonalization often complain of feelings of tiredness and hypersomnia, which in rare cases are severe enough to merit a differential diagnosis with a sleep disorder. In particular, recent evidence suggests that depersonalization is a common, if not invariable, symptom in patients with a sleep disorder known as Kleine–Levin syndrome (KLS). The latter is a fairly rare condition whose main symptoms are periodic hypersomnia accompanied by cognitive and behavioural disturbances. Eighty-one per cent of cases start during the second decade (median age of onset is 15), and there is a preponderance of male cases (68%). The condition should be kept in mind with young adults suffering from severe, intermittent depersonalization associated with hypersomnia. Indeed, a recent systematic review of 168 previously published cases diagnosed with KLS found that the vast majority of them had complained before of severe depersonalization and derealization, with some describing these symptoms as more noticeable and incapacitating than hypersomnia itself. In fact, some patients "questioned the existence of primary genuine hypersomnia and preferred to focus on an intense feeling of unreality which was so unpleasant that they tried to sleep to get away from it" (Landtblom *et al.*, 2003, p. 366). Similar findings came out of a survey on 108 new consecutive cases with KLS (Arnulf *et al.*, 2008). It was found that all patients complained of a variety of overlapping subjective experiences highly suggestive of depersonalization. For example, 81% complained of feeling as if they were in a dream ("things seemed hazy, foggy"), 63% were classified as suffering from 'derealization'; and 52% from a feeling of disconnection between the mind and the body. These symptoms were described as constant during the whole duration of each episode (Arnulf *et al.*, 2008). A summary of one case seen by the author, gives a good idea of the typical presenting complaints, which should raise suspicion of the condition.

The patient is a 26-year-old male with a 5-year history of recurrent episodes of severe depersonalization and concomitant severe hypersomnia. At the beginning of each episode, depersonalization was always the first symptom to be noticed by the patient, which he described as a feeling of being emotionally numb, and as if his body did not belong to him. Additionally, he reported that his surroundings seemed unreal. Such symptoms were typically experienced continuously for the duration of each episode, which lasted usually from 2 weeks to a month.

In addition to depersonalization, he complained of feeling constantly tired, and would sleep approximately 15–18 hours a day. However, he found his sleep non-restoring and experienced frequent nightmares.

His parents stated that during each episode he looked spaced out, sleepy, withdrawn and extremely irritable. Another prominent feature was a severe cognitive and attentional impairment, which would make it impossible for him to function. He claimed to be unable to read, have a conversation, watch television, cook or even walk his dog. He also claimed to be unable to experience hunger, and to lose his sense of smell or taste. Although he did not eat more than usual during the episodes, his parents stated that he would eat things he did not normally like. After running its natural course, each episode dissipated rapidly over the course of 1 or 2 days.

A brain MRI was found to be normal. An EEG carried out during one of the episodes showed generalized slowing.

Previous treatments with antidepressants, based on the assumption that he was suffering from depression, had not been effective.

In other cases seen by the author, depersonalization precedes the onset of hypersomnia, and cognitive impairment, and often remains as a residual condition for days or even weeks after the other symptoms have remitted.

REFERENCES

Arnulf, I., Zeitzer, J. M., File, J., Farber, N., Mignot, E. (2005). Kleine–Levin syndrome: a systematic review of 186 cases in the literature. *Brain*, **128**, 2763–2776.

Arnulf, I., Lin, L., Gadoth, N. *et al.* (2008). Kleine–Levin syndrome: a systematic study of 108 patients. *Annals of Neurology*, **63**, 482–493.

Baker, D., Hunter, E., Lawrence, E. *et al.* (2003). Depersonalisation disorder: clinical features of 204 cases. *British Journal of Psychiatry*, **182**, 428–433.

Blau, J. N. (1992). Classical migraine: Symptoms between visual aura and headache onset. *Lancet*, **340**, 355–356.

Brock, S., Wiesel, B. (1942). Derealization and depersonalization: their occurrence in organic and psychogenic states. *Diseases of the Nervous System*, **3**, 139–149.

Cahill, C. M., Murphy, K. C. (2004). Migraine and depersonalization disorder. *Cephalalgia*, **24**, 686–687.

Chong, S. A. (1995). Derealisation following head injury: a case report. *Singapore Medical Journal*, **36**, 568–569.

Cox, B. J., Swinson, R. P. (2002). Instrument to assess depersonalization-derealization in panic disorder. *Depression and Anxiety*, **5**, 172–175.

Davidson, K. (1964). Episodic depersonalisation: observations on 7 patients. *British Journal of Psychiatry*, **110**, 505–513.

Devinsky, O., Luciano, D. (1991). Psychic phenomena in partial seizures. *Seminars in Neurology*, **11**, 100–109.

Devinsky, O., Putnam, F., Grafman, J., Bromfield, E., Theodore, W. H. (1989). Dissociative states and epilepsy. *Neurology*, **39**, 835–840.

Devinsky, O., Feldmann, E., Bromfield, E., Emoto, S., Raubertas, R. (1991). Structured interview for partial seizures: clinical phenomenology and diagnosis. *Journal of Epilepsy*, **4**, 107–116.

Dietl, T., Bien, C., Urbach, H., Elger, C., Kurthen, M. (2005). Episodic depersonalization in focal epilepsy. *Epilepsy and Behaviour*, **7**, 311–315.

Frank, D. B. (1934). Depersonalizationserscheinungen bei Hirnerkrankungen. *Zeitschrift für die Gesamnte Neurologie und Psychiatrie*, **149**, 563–582.

Griesinger, W. (1868–69). Über einige epileptoide Zustände. *Archiv für Psychiatrie und Nervenkrankheiten*, **1**, 320–333.

Grigsby, J. (1986). Depersonalization following minor closed head injury. *The International Journal of Clinical Neuropsychology*, **8**, 65–68.

Grigsby, J. P., Johnston, C. L. (1989). Depersonalization, vertigo and Menière's disease. *Psychological Reports*, **64**, 527–534.

Grigsby, J., Kaye, K. (1993). Incidence and correlates of depersonalization following head trauma. *Brain Injury*, **7**, 507–513.

Haug, K. (1936). *Die Störungen des Persönlichkeitsbewusstseins und verwandte Entfremdungserlebnisse: eine klinische un psychologische Studie.* Stuttgart: Ferdinand Enke Verlag.

Heuyer, M. M. G., Dublineau, J. (1932). Syndrôme de dépersonnalisation chez un encéphalitique. *Annales Médico-Psychologiques,* **90,** 204–207.

Heuyer, G., Serin, M. (1920). Syndrôme de dépersonnalisation consécutif à une encéphalite épidémique. *L'Éncéphale,* **25,** 125–128.

Hoffer, M. E., Balough, B. J., Gottshall, K. R. (2007). Posttraumatic balance disorders. *International Tinnitus Journal,* **13,** 69–72.

Hunter, E. C., Phillips, M. L., Chalder, T., Sierra, M., David, A. S. (2003). Depersonalisation disorder: a cognitive-behavioural conceptualisation. *Behaviour Research and Therapy,* **41,** 1451–1467.

Jackson, H. (1889). On a particular variety of epilepsy ('intellectual aura'), one case with symptoms of organic brain disease. *Brain,* **11,** 179–207.

Jáuregui-Renaud, K., Sang, F. Y., Gresty, M. A., Green, D. A., Bronstein, A. M (2008). Depersonalisation/derealisation symptoms and updating orientation in patients with vestibular disease. *Journal of Neurology, Neurosurgery and Psychiatry,* **79,** 276–283.

Kanemoto, K. (1997). Periictal Capgras syndrome after clustered ictal fear: depth-electroencephalogram study. *Epilepsia,* **38,** 847–850.

Kew, J., Wright, A., Halligan, P. W. (1998). Somesthetic aura: the experience of "Alice in Wonderland". *Lancet,* **351,** 1934.

Krishaber, M. (1873). *De la Névropathie Cérébro-Cardiaque.* Paris: Masson.

Kunkel, R., S. (2005). Migraine aura without headache: benign, but a diagnosis of exclusion. *Cleveland Clinic Journal of Medicine,* **72,** 529–534.

Lambert, M. V., Sierra, M., Phillips, M. L., David, A. S. (2002). The spectrum of organic depersonalization: a review plus four new cases. *Journal of Neuropsychiatry and Clinical Neuroscience,* **14,** 141–154.

Landtblom, A. M., Dige, N., Schwerdt, K., Säfström, P., Granérus, G. (2003). Short-term memory dysfunction in Kleine–Levin syndrome. *Acta Neurologica Scandinavica,* **108,** 363–367.

Lawton, G., Baker, G. A., Brown, R. J. (2008). Comparison of two types of dissociation in epileptic and nonepileptic seizures. *Epilepsy and Behavior,* **13,** 333–336.

Lenggenhager, B., Smith, S. T., Blanke, O. (2006). Functional and neural mechanisms of embodiment: importance of the vestibular system and the temporal parietal junction. *Reviews in the Neurosciences,* **17,** 643–657.

Locatelli, M., Bellodi, L., Perna, G., Scarone, S. EEG power modifications in panic disorder during a temporolimbic activation task: relationships with temporal lobe clinical symptomatology (1993). *The Journal of Neuropsychiatry and Clinical Neurosciences,* **5,** 409–414.

Mayer-Gross, W. (1935). On depersonalisation. *British Journal of Medical Psychology,* **15,** 103–122.

Paulig, M., Böttger, S., Somme, R. M., Prosiegel, M. (1998). Depersonalisations-syndrom nach erworbener Hirnschädigung. *Nervenarzt,* **69,** 1100–1106.

Pelletier, G., Legendre-Roberge, J., Boileau, B., Geoffroy, G., Léveillé, J. (1995). Case study: dreamy state and temporal lobe dysfunction in a migrainous adolescent. *Journal of the American Academy of Child and Adolescent Psychiatry,* **34,** 297–301.

Persinger, M. A., Makarec, K. (1993). Complex partial epileptic signs as a continuum from normals to epileptics: normative data and clinical populations. *Journal of Clinical Psychology*, **49**, 33–45.

Pick, A. (1909). Zur Pathologie des Ich Bewusstseins. *Archiv für Psychiatrie und Nervenkrankheiten*, **38**, 22–23.

Phillips, M. L., Sierra, M. (2003). Depersonalization disorder: a functional neuroanatomical perspective. *Stress*, **6**, 157–165.

Podoll, K. (2005). Migraine Aura Foundation. http:/www.migraine-aura.org/content/e27891/e26585/e26706/index_en.html.

Podoll, K., Ebel, H. (1998). Halluzinationen der Körpervergrößerung bei der Migräne. *Fortschritte der Neurologie-Psychiatrie*, **66**, 259–270.

Roth, M., Harper, M. (1962). Temporal lobe epilepsy and the phobic anxiety depersonalisation syndrome. *Comprehensive Psychiatry*, **3**, 215–226.

Sacks, O. (1992). *Migraine*, 2nd edn. Reading, Berkshire: Picador. Cox & Wyman Ltd.

Sang, F. Y., Jáuregui-Renaud, K., Green, D. A., Bronstein, A. M., Gresty, M. A. (2006). Depersonalisation/derealisation symptoms in vestibular disease. *Journal of Neurology, Neurosurgery and Psychiatry*, **77**, 760–766.

Schilder, P. (1935). *The Image and Appearance of the Human Body*. London: Kegan Paul.

Sierra, M., Berrios, G. E. (2000). The Cambridge Depersonalization Scale: a new instrument for the measurement of depersonalization. *Psychiatry Research*, **93**, 153–164.

Shorvon, H. J. (1946). The depersonalisation syndrome. *Proceedings of the Royal Society of Medicine*, **39**, 779–792.

Silberman, E. K., Post, R. M., Nurnberger, J., Theodore, W., Boulenger, J. P. (1985). Transient sensory, cognitive and affective phenomena in affective illness: a comparison with complex partial epilepsy. *British Journal of Psychiatry*, **146**, 81–89.

Simeon, D., Knutelska, M., Nelson, D., Guralnik, O. (2003). Feeling unreal: a depersonalization disorder update of 117 cases. *The Journal of Clinical Psychiatry*, **64**, 990–997.

Ströhle, A., Kümpfel, T., Sonntag, A. (2000). Paroxetine for depersonalization associated with multiple sclerosis. *American Journal of Psychiatry*, **157**, 150.

Todd, J. (1963). The syndrome of Alice in Wonderland. *Canadian Medical Association Journal*, **73**, 701–704.

Toni, C., Cassano, G. B., Perugi, G., Murri, L. *et al.* (1996). Psychosensorial and related phenomena in panic disorder and in temporal lobe epilepsy. *Comprehensive Psychiatry*, **37**, 125–133.

Viviani, R., Berrios, G. E. (1996). 'On the pathology of the consciousness of the self' (by Pick, A.). *History of Psychiatry*, **7**, 319–332.

7

Depersonalization and culture

Introduction

As discussed in Chapter 2, a comparison of symptom profiles of historical and modern cases of depersonalization disorder suggests that depersonalization is a stable clinical phenomenon, whose manifestations seem impervious enough to cultural and historical influences (Sierra and Berrios, 2001). Surprisingly enough, however, the prevalence of the condition shows substantial variation across studies, and at least in psychiatric in-patients, has been reported as ranging from 7% to 80% (Hunter *et al.*, 2004). The cause of such wide variation is unknown. It could stem from differences in the criteria used to detect cases (including the lack of validated and standardised scales until recently); different nosological composition of the groups studied (depersonalization seems over-represented as a comorbid condition in certain diagnostic categories such as anxiety or depression); or transcultural differences. Interestingly enough, research on 'dissociative disorders' has also revealed a similarly wide range of prevalence amongst psychiatric patients. In this regard, it has been suggested that such differences reflect diagnostic biases rather than genuine prevalence differences (Friedl *et al.*, 2000). Some intriguing observations, however, would seem to point to genuine differences in the prevalence of dissociative symptoms (including depersonalization) across different cultures. For example, it has been reported that the prevalence of DSM-IV or ICD-10 'dissociative disorders' seems so low amongst Indian psychiatric in-patients as to cast doubt on the clinical relevance of this diagnostic category in India (Das and Saxena, 1991; Alexander *et al.*, 1997). Parikh *et al.* (1981), for example, used the Dixon depersonalization scale to screen a sample of 288 Indian psychiatric in-patients and found that only 7.6% reported depersonalization symptoms. In contrast, another study in which a similar self-rating questionnaire was used, found that, in a sample of 100 American psychiatric in-patients, 40% endorsed at least five features of depersonalization (Noyes *et al.*, 1977).

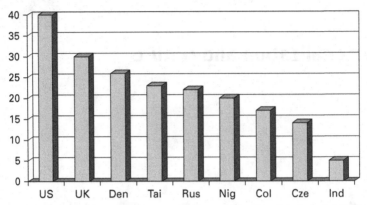

Fig. 7.1. Prevalence of derealization in patients with schizophrenia in the WHO Pilot Study (percentage of patients reporting the symptom). Abbreviations: Den = Denmark, Tai = Taiwan, Rus = Russia, Nig = Nigeria, Col = Colombia, Cze = Czech Republic, Ind = India

A similar trend can also be observed in the prevalence of 'derealization' as reported by the International Pilot Study of Schizophrenia (World Health Organization, 1973). As can be seen in Fig. 7.1, whilst the highest prevalence of 'derealization' in schizophrenia patients was found in the US and Western Europe (US 40%, UK 30%, Denmark 26%), the lowest was found in Asia, Latin America and Eastern Europe (Colombia 17%, Czech Republic 16%, India 5%).

A recent survey carried out in mainland China, using the Chinese version of the Dissociative Experiences Scale, found that the prevalence of depersonalization symptoms was only 1.6% amongst 304 out-patients attending a Mental Health Centre (Xiao *et al.*, 2006a). The authors also administered the Dissociative Disorders Interview Schedule to establish the prevalence of dissociative disorders. In addition to the out-patients group the author also assessed 423 psychiatric in-patients and 618 factory workers. No cases in the out-patients sample met criteria for depersonalization disorder, whilst only one case was found in each of the other two groups. Such prevalence figures are substantially lower than those found in a similar study carried out in Canada (Xiao *et al.*, 2006b).

Similarly, a study comparing the frequency of depersonalization in psychiatric in-patients from the UK ($n = 31$), Spain ($n = 68$), and Colombia ($n = 41$), found the prevalence of depersonalization symptoms to be significantly lower in the Colombian patients, irrespective of diagnosis (see Fig. 7.2). No significant differences were found on measures of depression, anxiety, or dissociative dimensions other than depersonalization (Sierra *et al.*, 2006). Given that Colombian patients had a similar or slightly higher educational level compared with that of British and Spanish patients, respectively, it is unlikely that their low scores on depersonalization were an artefact of poor education or

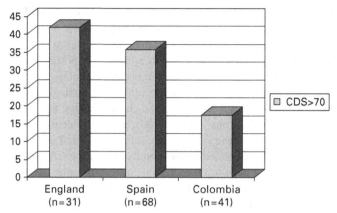

Fig. 7.2. Percentage of patients suffering comorbid depersonalization syndrome (score >70 on the Cambridge Depersonalization Scale) (taken from Sierra *et al.*, 2006).

linguistic competence. Also, the fact that all administered scales in this study were self-rated excludes the possibility of diagnostic biases. All in all, the findings of this and previous studies seem to suggest the existence of true cultural effects, which would seem to make depersonalization a rarer occurrence in Asian and Latin American countries as compared to Western Europe and North America.

In view of the fact that depersonalization entails an anomalous experience of the self, we have previously hypothesized that cultural influences on how the self is construed, may be of relevance to explain prevalence differences across cultures (Sierra *et al.*, 2006). Indeed, it has been established that the concept and experience of the self can vary considerably across cultures, and it would seem that this is greatly determined by variations on a dimension known as 'individualism–collectivism' (Markus and Kitayama, 1991). In short, 'individualism' refers to the degree to which a person experiences himself or herself as an autonomous and independent being: the bearer of an invariable set of attributes not affected by social context. The term 'collectivism', in contrast, views the self as a permeable entity, in constant interdependency with the surrounding context, so that here it is the 'other' or rather, the 'self-in-relation-to-other' that is central in individual experience (Triandis, 2001; Markus and Kitayama, 1991). It has been established empirically that, whilst the 'West' as a whole is characterized by highly individualistic cultures, Asia, Africa and most Latin American countries are predominantly collectivistic (Triandis *et al.*, 1984, 2001, 2002).

Emerging evidence suggests that individualism–collectivism can exert a far-reaching shaping influence on cognition and emotions. For example, an interesting study compared European American and Chinese children on the content of their autobiographical memories and self-descriptions elicited by means of open-ended questions. It was found that, whilst American children "often provided elaborate and detailed memories focusing on their own roles, preferences, and feelings; they also frequently described themselves in terms of personal attributes, abstract dispositions, and inner traits in a positive light. Chinese children provided relatively skeletal accounts of past experiences that centred on social interactions and daily routines, and they often described themselves in terms of social roles, context-specific characteristics, and other behaviours in a neutral or modest tone" (Wang, 2004, p. 3). Similar studies on autobiographical memory comparing adults from collectivistic and individualistic cultural backgrounds have yielded similar results (Wang, 2006, 2008). In a fascinating experiment intended to test the effect of culture on context-related biases at a perceptual level, Kitayama *et al.* (2003) were able to show that, as compared with Asian participants, American subjects showed a systematic perceptual bias against context-related information. In short, subjects were shown a square frame with a vertical line inside. They were then presented with another square frame of either the same or different size and were asked to draw a line inside so that it was: (a) identical in length to the original ('absolute task'); or (b) so that the line/square proportion was reproduced ('relative task'). As predicted, it was found that, whilst Japanese participants were more accurate in the 'relative task' (a task which required the use of context-related information), Americans performed better in the 'absolute task'. A subsequent functional magnetic resonance imaging (fMRI) study carried out as subjects performed an adapted version of the above tasks, found a higher activation in attention relevant areas such as frontal and parietal regions, when subjects performed a non-culturally preferred task. For example, Asian subjects showed more activation in attentional related areas when performing the 'absolute' task. Such a pattern of activation probably reflects higher cognitive effort, and control demands over working memory and attention, when individuals perform cognitive tasks, which have little 'ecological' value in their respective culture (Hedden *et al.*, 2008). Further studies using psycho-physiological measures such as event-related potentials have provided additional backing to these findings and show the extent to which cultural influences seem to shape neural responses associated with attentional control and perception (Lewis *et al.*, 2008).

Although the effects of 'individualism–collectivism' on psychopathology remains a poorly explored area, it would seem that highly 'individualistic' cultures confer vulnerability to conditions characterized by alienation feelings (Draguns and Tanaka-Matsumi, 2003). In this regard, it would seem plausible that individualistic cultures confer vulnerability to depersonalization, and that prevalence difference across cultures might be accounted for by variations on the 'individualism–collectivism' spectrum (Sierra *et al.*, 2006). In order to test this idea, we carried out a comprehensive systematic review of published empirical studies on panic disorder in which the frequency of depersonalization/derealization during panic attacks was reported (Sierra-Siegert and David, 2007). The reasons for choosing panic disorder were severalfold:

(1) The large amount of empirical studies carried out in the last two decades.
(2) The fact that panic attacks are known and recognizable in most cultures (McNally, 1994; Amering and Katschnig, 1990).
(3) Both DSM-IV and ICD-10 consider depersonalization as one of the constituent symptoms of a panic attack.

It was predicted that panic disorder patients from 'Western cultures' would show, as a group, a higher frequency of depersonalization than patients from non-Western cultures; and that a significant correlation would be found between the frequency of depersonalization and the corresponding 'individualism' score for each country, as determined by Hofstede's classical study (Hofstede, 1991). Hoftstede's 'individualism' scores have been used widely in sociological research, and were originally derived from a worldwide research on values at the work place in more than 71 countries (Hofstede, 1991, 2001). Individualism scores are available for about 55 countries and range from 5 in the case of Guatemala, to 91 in the case of the US. Although the original scores were generated in 1973, subsequent research has been able to validate and replicate the original findings (Merritt, 2000; Schimmack et al., 2005).

Out of a total of 356 screened papers, 50 selected studies reported on panic symptoms from patient samples of 21 different countries. The range of reported frequency for depersonalization was 75.8% (US) to 5% (Turkey); the overall mean was 45.6% ± 17.4% (Sierra-Siegert and David, 2007).

In keeping with previous findings, it was found that the prevalence of 'depersonalization' was significantly lower in Asian and Latin American countries, as compared with North America, Western Europe, Australia and New Zealand. Interestingly, the frequency of 'fear of losing control' was also significantly lower in non-Western countries (see Table 7.1).

As predicted, there was a highly significant correlation between 'individualism' and 'depersonalization' (see Fig. 7.3). In keeping with such an association, a recent epidemiological study on the prevalence of depersonalization in the German general population found that the prevalence of clinically relevant depersonalization was higher in West Germany as compared with eastern regions previously under communist regime (Michal et al., 2009). Given that such a difference remained after controlling for potentially confounding socio-demographic variables, the authors ascribed it to the fact that West Germany is still characterized by higher levels of 'individualism' than former socialist East Germany (Martin et al., 2000). Interestingly enough, as can be seen in Fig. 7.1, the Czech republic, which at the time of the WHO study (1973) was a communist state, also yielded a surprisingly low prevalence of derealization as compared with other European countries at the time.

Table 7.1. Individualism Index and frequency of panic symptoms across Western and non-Western countries.

	Western countries ($n = 37$)	Non-Western countries ($n = 13$)	Mann-Whitney Z and P values
Individualism score	80.4 (14.1)	37.9 (9.2)	$Z = -5.02\ P < 0.0001$
Depersonalization	52.6 (12.3)	25.6 (14.0)	$Z = -4.7\ P < 0.0001$
Fear of losing control	67.0 (17.9)	35.8 (18.0)	$Z = -2.91\ P = 0.004$
Palpitations	84.7 (6.80)	87.3 (9.0)	$Z = -0.92\ P = 0.35$
Shortness of breath	69.3 (12.6)	74.8 (14.6)	$Z = -1.32\ P = 0.18$
Chest pain	55.9 (12.3)	58.8 (22.8)	$Z = -0.02\ P = 0.98$
Choking	49.2 (15.0)	48.7 (25.8)	$Z = -0.55\ P = 0.58$
Chills/hot flushes	63.5 (13.8)	51.8 (18.1)	$Z = -1.53\ P = 0.12$
Sweating	70.1 (11.9)	55.6 (20.6)	$Z = -1.44\ P = 0.14$
Paresthesias	49.5 (16.2)	51.0 (19.5)	$Z = -0.08\ P = 0.93$
Trembling	69.4 (15.6)	54.2 (22.8)	$Z = -1.6\ P = 0.093$
Dizziness	72.4 (16.5)	59.42 (17.4)	$Z = -1.2\ P = 0.22$
Nausea	45.6 (11.1)	45.4 (19.9)	$Z = -0.66\ P = 0.50$
Fear of dying	64.4 (15.4)	72.8 (21.7)	$Z = -1.4\ P = 0.27$

The 'Western' group was composed of the US, Canada, Denmark, Sweden, Switzerland, Germany, France, the Netherlands, Italy, Spain, Portugal, Australia and New Zealand. The non-Western group was composed of Japan, South Korea, India, Iran, Thailand, Turkey and Russia.
From Sierra-Siegert, M., David, A. S. (2007).

In addition to the correlation between depersonalization and individualism the study on panic symptoms across cultures also found similarly high correlations between 'individualism' and 'fear of losing control'; and between the latter and 'depersonalization' (Sierra-Siegert and David, 2007). Such findings were interpreted as suggesting that 'feelings of lack of control' might be a relevant experience mediating the effects of individualism on depersonalization. Interestingly, both 'depersonalization' and 'fear of losing control' have been found to correlate in other anxiety disorder studies (Meuret *et al.*, 2006; Kenardy *et al.*, 1992). For example, in a factor analysis study on 390 outpatients with anxiety disorders, researchers obtained a factor containing these two symptoms only, which was labelled 'psychological threat' (Kenardy *et al.*, 1992). This association between 'fear of losing control' and 'depersonalization' in panic disorder patients lends support to the view that perceived lack of control and related cognitive attributions may have a role in the triggering and maintenance of depersonalization responses (Hunter *et al.*, 2003). Indeed, unlike the case with 'the fight or flight' response, threats capable of triggering depersonalization are typically characterized by a feeling of not being in control (Sierra and Berrios, 1998). It is plausible to assume, in this respect, that the

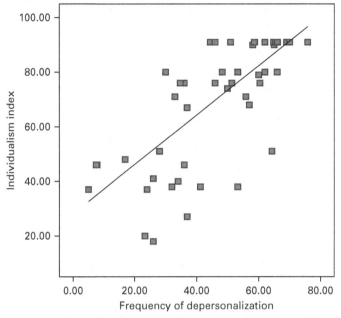

Fig. 7.3. Correlation between individualism scores and frequency of depersonalization/ derealization during panic attacks (from Sierra-Siegert, M., David, A. S., 2007).

sudden onset of an unprovoked panic attack could constitute in itself such 'no-control'-perceived threat. In support of this idea, it has been found that panic disorder patients who depersonalize have an earlier onset and a more severe course of the disease than those who don't depersonalize (Cassano *et al.*, 1989; Katerndahl and Talamantes, 2000; Marquez *et al.*, 2001). Moreover, recent findings suggest that the experience of panic can indeed be a mediating mechanism capable of triggering dissociative responses during acute trauma (Bryant and Panasetis, 2005; Nixon *et al.*, 2004). In the same vein, it is likely that episodes of acute anxiety and 'no control feelings' could mediate experiences of depersonalization associated with the use of illicit drugs. In this regard, a study compared 40 cases of 'drug-induced depersonalization' with 122 cases of non-drug induced, and found that, whilst 90% of those in the drug-induced group admitted to a history of anxiety and/or panic attacks, only 29% in the non-drug group did (Medford *et al.*, 2003). It is clear, however, that the experience of panic is not sufficient to trigger depersonalization, given that it does not occur in a substantial proportion of patients. This suggests that, in addition to the intensity of the triggering stimulus situation (e.g. autonomic arousal), psychological and social dimensions of self-experience may also modulate a subjective 'threat detection' threshold. As reviewed in Chapter 4, research into potential predisposing factors for the occurrence of depersonalization during panic has not been conclusive. However, there is some evidence that patients who depersonalize during panic attacks may be characterized by more frequent emotional or sexual abuse in childhood, than those who don't experience depersonalization (McWilliams *et al.*, 2001).

Our findings suggest that, as compared with collectivistic societies, subjects from individualistic cultures are likely to experience more 'fear of loss of control' and 'depersonalization' during panic attacks. Interestingly enough, it has been found that individuals from individualistic societies are more 'self-absorbed' and have a more externalized locus of control, which makes them more sensitive to threat, to feelings of alienation and of not being in control (Smith, 1990; Roberts and Helson, 1997; Twenge and Zhang, 2004). In contrast, it would seem that a sense of belonging and shared values in relation to a cultural group provide individuals from collectivistic societies with a sense of 'implicit social support', whose protective effect to threat has been shown in the form of attenuated psychological and biological responses (blood pressure, heart rate, cortisol levels) to experimental stressful conditions (Taylor *et al.*, 2007; Shen *et al.*, 2004). Supporting the potential role of 'implicit support' as a protective factor against threat and depersonalization experiences, an epidemiological study explored the relationship between church attendance and prevalence of depersonalization in a community-based sample (Alderibigbe *et al.*, 2001). It was found that less frequent church attendance was associated with a higher frequency of reported depersonalization. Furthermore, the fact that strength of religious belief was not found to be relevant to the association suggests that "the social aspects of church attendance may be related to the decreased reports of dissociative symptoms" (p. 66).

At the level of the individual (as opposed to cultures), self-experience has also been shown to be influenced by both 'individualistic' and 'collectivistic' self-representations. It has been experimentally found that, as compared with people whose 'collective self' is threatened, those whose 'individual self' is threatened typically experience the threat as being more severe, experience a more negative mood and report more anger (Gaertner *et al.*, 1999).

It may be speculated that exposure to emotional abuse in childhood, a known predisposing factor to depersonalization in adulthood (Simeon *et al.*, 2001), may hinder the development of a representation of the self, which is grounded on an experience of group membership (i.e. collective self-representation). This would lead to a 'lopsided' self-representation, which overemphasizes its individualistic dimension and makes it hypersensitive to threat (i.e. self-representation independent of group membership) and to experiences of alienation and lack of control.

A recent study (Michal *et al.*, 2006) compared 20 patients with pathological depersonalization with a group of clinical controls on a measure of personality structure (German Narcissism Inventory). As compared with the control group, patients with depersonalization scored significantly higher on most items of a subscale named the 'threatened self', which addresses feelings of alienation, and of not being in control.

Although more research is needed in this area, it is clear that the study of 'individualism–collectivism' may prove valuable in the understanding of depersonalization predisposition.

REFERENCES

Aderibigbe, Y. A., Bloch, R. M., Walker, W. R. (2001). Prevalence of depersonalization and derealization experiences in a rural population. *Social Psychiatry and Psychiatry Epidemiology*, **36**, 63–69.

Alexander, P. J., Joseph, S., Das, A. (1997). Limited utility of ICD-10 and DSM-IV classification of dissociative and conversion disorders in India. *Acta Psychiatrica Scandinavica*, **95**, 177–182.

Amering, M., Katschnig, H. (1990). Panic attacks and panic disorder in cross-cultural perspective. *Psychiatric Annals*, **20**, 511–516.

Bryant, R. A., Panasetis, P. (2005). The role of panic in acute dissociative reactions following trauma. *British Journal of Clinical Psychology*, **44**, 489–494.

Cassano, G. B., Petracca, A., Perugi, G., Toni, C., Tundo, A., Roth, M. (1989). Derealization and panic attacks: a clinical evaluation on 150 patients with panic disorder/agoraphobia. *Comprehensive Psychiatry*, **30**, 5–12.

Das, P. S., Saxena, S. (1991). Classification of dissociative states in DSM-III-R and ICD-10 (1989 draft). A study of Indian out-patients. *British Journal of Psychiatry*, **159**, 425–427.

Draguns, J. G., Tanaka-Matsumi, J. (2003). Assessment of psychopathology across and within cultures: issues and findings. *Behavioral Research Therapy*, **41**, 755–776.

Friedl, M. C., Draijer, N., de Jonge, P. (2000). Prevalence of dissociative disorders in psychiatric in-patients: the impact of study characteristics. *Acta Psychiatrica Scandinavica*, **102**, 423–428.

Gaertner, L., Sedikides, C., Graetz, K. (1999). In search of self-definition: motivational primacy of the individual self, motivational primacy of the collective self, or contextual primacy? *Journal of Personality and Social Psychology*, **76**, 5–18.

Hedden, T., Ketay, S., Aron, A., Markus, H. R., Gabrieli, J. D. (2008). Cultural influences on neural substrates of attentional control. *Psychological Science*, **19**, 12–17.

Hofstede, G. (1991). *Cultures and Organizations: Software of the Mind*. London, UK: McGraw-Hill.

Hofstede, G. (2001). *Culture's Consequences, Comparing Values, Behaviors, Institutions, and Organizations, Across Nations*. Thousand Oaks, CA: Sage Publications.

Hunter, E. C., Phillips, M. L., Chalder, T., Sierra, M., David, A. S. (2003). Depersonalisation disorder: a cognitive-behavioural conceptualisation. *Behavioral Research Therapy*, **41**, 1451–1467.

Hunter, E. C., Sierra, M., David, A. S. (2004). The epidemiology of depersonalisation and derealisation: a systematic review. *Social Psychiatry and Psychiatry Epidemiology*, **39**, 9–18.

Lewis, R. S., Goto, S. G., Kong, L. L. (2008). Culture and context: East Asian American and European American differences in P3 event-related potentials and self-construal. *Personality and Social Psychology Bulletin*, **34**, 623–634.

Katerndahl, D. A., Talamantes, M. (2000). A comparison of persons with early- versus late-onset panic attacks. *Journal of Clinical Psychiatry*, **61**, 422–427.

Kenardy, J., Evans, L., Oei, T. P. (1992). The latent structure of anxiety symptoms in anxiety disorders. *American Journal of Psychiatry*, **149**, 1058–1061.

Kitayama, S., Duffy, S., Kawamura, T., Larsen, J. T. (2003). Perceiving an object and its context in different cultures: a cultural look at new look. *Psychological Science*, **14**, 201–206.

Markus, H. R., Kitayama, Sh. (1991). Culture and the self: implications for cognition, emotion, and motivation. *Psychological Review*, **98**, 224–253.

Marquez, M., Segui, J., Garcia, L., Canet, J., Ortiz, M. (2001). Is panic disorder with psychosensorial symptoms (depersonalization-derealization) a more severe clinical subtype? *Journal of Nervous and Mental Disease*, **189**, 332–335.

Martin, P., Grünendahl, M., Schmitt, M. (2000). Persönlichkeit, kognitive Leistungsfähigkeit und Gesundheit in Ost und West: Ergebnisse der Interdisziplinären Längsschnittstudie des Erwachsenenalters. *Zeitschrift für Gerontologie und Geriatrie*, **33**, 111–123.

McNally, R. J. (1994). *Panic Disorder: A Critical Analysis*. NY: The Guilford Press.

McWilliams, L. A., Cox, B. J., Enns, M. W. (2001). Trauma and depersonalization during panic attacks. *American Journal of Psychiatry*, **158**, 656–657.

Medford, N., Baker, D., Hunter, E. *et al.* (2003). Chronic depersonalization following illicit drug use: a controlled analysis of 40 cases. *Addiction*, **98**, 1731–1736.

Merritt, A. (2000). Culture in the cockpit: do Hofstede's dimensions replicate? *Journal of Cross-Cultural Psychology*, **31**, 283–301.

Meuret, A. E., White, K. S., Ritz, T., Roth, W. T., Hofmann, S. G., Brown, T. A. (2006). Panic attack symptom dimensions and their relationship to illness characteristics in panic disorder. *Journal of Psychiatry Research*, **40**, 520–527.

Michal, M., Kaufhold, J., Overbeck, G., Grabhorn, R. (2006). Narcissistic regulation of the self and interpersonal problems in depersonalized patients. *Psychopathology*, **39**, 192–198.

Michal, M., Wiltink, J., Subic-Wrana, C. *et al.* (2009). Prevalence, correlates and predictors of depersonalization experiences in the German general population. *Journal of Nervous and Mental Disease*, in press.

Nixon, R. D., Resick, P. A., Griffin, M. G. (2004). Panic following trauma: the etiology of acute posttraumatic arousal. *Journal of Anxiety Disorders*, **18**, 193–210.

Noyes, R., Hoenk, P. R., Kuperman, S., Slymen, D. J. (1977). Depersonalization in accident victims and psychiatric patients. *Journal of Nervous and Mental Disease*, **164**, 401–407.

Parikh, M. D., Sheth, A. S., Apte, J. S. (1981). Depersonalization: A phenomenological study in psychiatric patients. *Journal of Postgraduate Medicine*, **27**, 226–230.

Roberts, B. W., Helson, R. (1997). Changes in culture, changes in personality: the influence of individualism in a longitudinal study of women. *Journal of Personality and Social Psychology*, **72**, 641–651.

Schimmack, U., Oishi, S., Diener, E. (2005). Individualism: a valid and important dimension of cultural differences between nations. *Personality and Social Psychology Review*, **9**, 17–31.

Shen, B. J., Stroud, L. R., Niaura, R. (2004). Ethnic differences in cardiovascular responses to laboratory stress: a comparison between Asian and white Americans. *International Journal of Behavioral Medicine*, **11**, 181–186.

Sierra, M., Berrios, G. E. (1998). Depersonalization: neurobiological perspectives. *Biological Psychiatry*, **44**, 898–908.

Sierra, M., Berrios, G. E. (2000). The Cambridge Depersonalization Scale: a new instrument for the measurement of depersonalization. *Psychiatry Research*, **93**, 153–164.

Sierra, M., Berrios, G. E. (2001). The phenomenological stability of depersonalization: comparing the old with the new. *Journal of Nervous and Mental Disease*, **189**, 629–636.

Sierra, M., Baker, D., Medford, N., David, A. S. (2005). Unpacking the depersonalization syndrome: an exploratory factor analysis on the Cambridge Depersonalization Scale. *Psychological Medicine*, **35**, 1523–1532.

Sierra, M., Gomez, J., Molina, J. J., Luque, R., Muñoz, J. F., David, A. S. (2006). Depersonalization in psychiatric patients: a transcultural study. *Journal of Nervous and Mental Disease*, **194**, 356–361.

Sierra-Siegert, M., David, A. S. (2007). Depersonalization and individualism: the effect of culture on symptom profiles in panic disorder. *Journal of Nervous and Mental Disease*, **195**, 989–995.

Simeon, D., Guralnik, O., Schmeidler, J., Sirof, B., Knutelska, M. (2001). The role of childhood interpersonal trauma in depersonalization disorder. *American Journal of Psychiatry*, **158**, 1027–1033.

Smith, B. M. (1990). The measurement of narcissism in Asian, Caucasian and Hispanic American women. *Psychological Report*, **7**, 779–785.

Taylor, S. E., Welch, W. T., Kim, H. S., Sherman, D. K. (2007). Cultural differences in the impact of social support on psychological and biological stress responses. *Psychology of Science*, **18**, 831–837.

Triandis, H. C. (2001). Individualism-collectivism and personality. *Journal of Personality and Social Psychology*, **69**, 907–924.

Triandis, H. C., Suh, E. M. (2002). Cultural influences on personality. *Annual Reviews of Psychology*, **53**, 133–160.

Triandis, H. C., Marin, G., Lisansky, J., Betancourt, H. (1984). Simpatia as a cultural script for Hispanics. *Journal of Personality and Social Psychology*, **47**, 1363–1375.

Twenge, J. M., Zhang, L., Im, C. (2004). It's beyond my control: a cross-temporal meta-analysis of increasing externality in locus of control, 1960–2002. *Personality and Social Psychology Review*, **8**, 308–319.

Wang, Q. (2004). The emergence of cultural self-constructs: autobiographical memory and self-description in European American and Chinese children. *Developmental Psychology*, **40**, 3–15.

Wang, Q. (2006). Earliest recollections of self and others in European, American and Taiwanese young adults. *Psychological Science*, **17**, 708–714.

Wang, Q. (2008). Being American, being Asian: the bicultural self and autobiographical memory in Asian Americans. *Cognition*, **107**, 743–751.

World Health Organization (1973). *The International Pilot Study of Schizophrenia*, Vol 1. Geneva: WHO.

Xiao, Z., Yan, H., Wang, Z. *et al.* (2006a). Trauma and dissociation in China. *American Journal of Psychiatry*, **163**, 1388–1391.

Xiao, Z., Yan, H., Wang, Z. *et al.* (2006b). Dissociative experiences in China. *Journal of Trauma and Dissociation*, **7**, 23–38.

8

Towards a pharmacology of depersonalization

Introduction

Little is known about useful pharmacological treatments for depersonalization disorder, and the condition has been generally considered refractory to most medications. There are historical reports of the use of barbiturates, amphetamines, neuroleptics, etc. all with no consistent benefit. Fortunately, this bleak and rather hopeless scenario has gradually begun to change during the last decade. Indeed, a number of studies involving both challenge and therapeutic trials suggest that a few key neurotransmitter systems may be of particular relevance to the pathophysiology of depersonalization, and a few promising medications have been identified.

Depersonalization and serotonin

Evidence pointing to a serotonergic involvement in depersonalization comes from 'challenge' studies, as well as from therapeutic trials with serotonergic antidepressants.

'Challenge' studies

A number of substances with predominant serotonergic effects have been reported to induce depersonalization-like experiences and suggest that serotonergic mechanisms are important to the neurobiology of depersonalization.

The most relevant study in this regard was carried out using the 5-HT2c agonist meta-chlorophenylpiperazine (m-CPP) in an attempt to induce depersonalization in 67 subjects under double-blind placebo-controlled conditions (Simeon *et al.*, 1995). It was found that, when challenged with m-CPP, 18% of the participants experienced depersonalization or derealization. However, a potential confounder with m-CPP is that it can induce panic attacks, which as is known, frequently trigger depersonalization symptoms. Indeed, the authors found a striking correlation of 0.7 between the induction of depersonalization and the development of panic symptoms, which makes it unclear whether the induction of depersonalization was a direct effect of a serotonergic challenge, or was indirectly mediated by an ensuing panic attack.

Psilocybin, a powerful serotonergic agonist on $5\text{-HT}_{2A/1A}$ receptors, has also been found to induce depersonalization in a dose-dependent manner under placebo-controlled conditions. Interestingly enough, it was found that the presence of depersonalization correlated with subjective feelings of time distortion and impairment in working memory (Wittmann et al., 2007). Such a relationship between depersonalization and distorted time experience had been noticed in previous studies focusing on the effects of cannabis on cognition (Melges et al., 1970). In fact, cannabis has been shown to be a potent inducer of depersonalization experiences (see below). Although the main pharmacological effects of cannabis are mediated through cannabinoid receptors, it is also known to severely disrupt serotonergic neurotransmission. For example, functional electrophysiological studies have shown that activation of pre-synaptic cannabinoid CB_1 receptors results in decreased 5-HT release in the neocortex (Nakazi et al., 2000). It would seem, in fact, that most of cannabis's effects on cognition and perception are mediated by its disruptive effect on serotonergic neurotransmission (Russo et al., 2005; Hill et al., 2006) and it is likely that its ability to induce depersonalization is related to this effect. One study found that cannabis smoking, but not placebo smoking, was able to produce depersonalization feelings in 62% of 35 healthy subjects (Mathew et al., 1993). The intensity of depersonalization reached a peak after 30 minutes and returned to the baseline after 120 minutes. A comparison of the effects of high vs. low potency cannabis cigarettes established that the ability of cannabis to induce depersonalization was dose dependent rather than an idiosyncratic response to the drug.

Therapeutic effects of serotonergic antidepressants

Several reports on the use of serotonin-selective reuptake inhibitor (SSRI) antidepressants on single cases or small series of patients with depersonalization disorder have suggested that these medications have a promising role in the treatment of this condition. For example, a group of researchers used SSRIs on a sample of eight consecutive patients with long-standing prominent depersonalization symptoms, most of which met criteria for depersonalization disorder (Hollander et al., 1990). The authors noted high levels of comorbidity with anxiety disorders or obsessive compulsive disorder, and reported that the presence of either seemed to predict a better response to SSRIs. Other retrospective accounts of the effectiveness of SSRIs on depersonalization disorder were less conclusive and suggestive of only marginal beneficial effects

(Simeon *et al.*, 2003). Furthermore, this initial promise of SSRIs has not been supported by a double-blind study, in which fluoxetine was not found more effective than placebo in 54 patients with DSM-IV Depersonalization Disorder (Simeon *et al.*, 2004). However, in line with the earlier study discussed above (Hollander *et al.*, 1990), it was found that those patients with a comorbid diagnosis of depressive or anxiety disorder tended to fare better on fluoxetine than on placebo. Thus, in nine patients who had an additional diagnosis of anxiety disorder, improvement of the anxiety condition was invariably associated with an improvement in depersonalization. However, those experiencing some improvement clarified that the depersonalization feelings had not really changed but that 'they seemed somehow to take less notice or be less bothered by them' (Simeon *et al.*, 2004).

In another attempt to test serotonergic mechanisms in depersonalization, researchers carried out a double-blind, cross-over trial to compare the efficacy of clomipramine (a serotonin-selective tricyclic antidepressant) and desipramine (a norepinephrine-selective tricyclic antidepressant), on eight patients with depersonalization disorder during an 8-week trial. Of seven subjects who completed the clomipramine phase of the trial, two showed significant improvement in depersonalization (Simeon *et al.*, 1998). Although one of the latter responded to both medications, she claimed that clomipramine had a more substantial effect on depersonalization. Of interest, none of the responders had depression, but one had a comorbid diagnosis of social phobia.

In view of the above results it has to be concluded that the use of SSRIs or clomipramine as sole medications are not indicated for the treatment of depersonalization disorder. It is possible, however, that their use on patients with prominent anxiety and depression symptoms may result in improved tolerance of depersonalization symptoms.

Another group of medications, which are relevant to the putative role of serotonin on depersonalization, are the monoamino oxidase inhibitors (MAOIs). The latter impair the breakdown of serotonin as well as norepinephrine and dopamine. Although there are no systematic studies on the effects of MAOIs on depersonalization disorder, they have been found useful in the treatment of a type of depression characterized by depersonalization and anxiety (Davidson *et al.*, 1989). That this effect might be serotonin mediated is hinted at by the observation that pre-treatment with MAOIs can attenuate or abolish the effects of LSD (Resnick *et al.*, 1964). The latter is known to act mainly on the serotonin system and to induce depersonalization symptoms (Sedman and Kenna, 1964).

Further support for an underlying relationship between depersonalization disorder and anxiety disorders comes from anecdotal reports showing that clonazepam, either on its own or in association with SSRIs has beneficial effects on depersonalization disorder (Lambert *et al.*, 2000; Sachdev, 2002). Stein *et al.* carried out a detailed pharmacological investigation on a patient with a 6-year history of continuous depersonalization (i.e. depersonalization disorder) and no history of anxiety or affective disorders (Stein and Uhde, 1989). A challenge phase of the study revealed that the administration of caffeine, but not of placebo, produced a consistent increase in depersonalization, and also triggered panic attacks which the patient had never experienced before. It was also found that the single-blind administration of clonazepam, but not of carbamazepine, brought about a dramatic improvement of depersonalization. Furthermore, a re-challenge with caffeine while under the effects of clonazepam failed to increase depersonalization intensity.

Depersonalization and glutamate

Other researchers have suggested that excitatory amino acids such as glutamate might be relevant to the pathophysiology of depersonalization and dissociation in general (Chambers *et al.*, 1999). For example, subanaesthetic doses of ketamine, whose effects might be mediated through increased glutamate release, can induce many of the subjective experiences characteristic of depersonalization, including a sense of detachment and emotional numbing (Krystal *et al.*, 1994). Interestingly enough, a recent fMRI study found that subjects with 'ketamine-induced depersonalization' showed abnormalities in the processing of emotional stimuli, which were similar to those previously reported in patients with depersonalization disorder (Abel *et al.*, 2003). Thus, subjects with 'ketamine-induced depersonalization' and those with depersonalization disorder have shown a lack of activity in limbic areas and hyperactivity in prefrontal cortical regions that may be important for mood regulation (Phillips *et al.*, 2001; Abel *et al.*, 2003). It is believed that 'ketamine-induced depersonalization' is mediated by increased glutamate release in response to NMDA receptor blockade, with a consequent excess of glutamate activity at non-NMDA glutamate receptors (Krystal *et al.*, 1994). In keeping with this hypothesis, it has been found that pre-treatment with lamotrigine, a drug reported to inhibit glutamate release by action at the presynaptic membrane, attenuates the effects of ketamine on conscious experience and cognition (Anand *et al.*, 2000).

In order to test the hypothesis that depersonalization is glutamate mediated, Sierra *et al.* (2003) carried out a small double-blind, cross-over, placebo-controlled trial on nine patients with depersonalization disorder. Unfortunately, the results failed to show any positive effects of lamotrigine when taken as a sole medication. In spite of these negative results, two open-label trials using lamotrigine as an add-on medication with antidepressants, particularly of the SSRI type, suggest that 50%–70% of patients with depersonalization disorder experience varying degrees of improvement (Sierra *et al.*, 2001, 2006). Although these two studies did not control for placebo effects, it is worth noticing that double-blind studies have found negligible placebo effects in depersonalization disorder (Simeon *et al.*, 2004; Sierra *et al.*, 2003). Such findings suggest that, rather than acting on its own, lamotrigine works better as an add-on therapy with SSRI antidepressants. This possibility would not be surprising, in view of the circumstantial evidence reviewed earlier, which points to an involvement of both serotonergic and glutamatergic mechanisms in depersonalization. If that is indeed the case, it may be that successful pharmacological interventions need to target both neurotransmitter systems. It is clear that these promising results warrant further, more rigorous research.

Depersonalization and the opioid system

Ample evidence supports the view that the endogenous opioid system is involved in the regulation of emotional and behavioural responses to stress (Cohen *et al.*, 1983). Indeed, activation of this system has been shown to lead to increased pain threshold, suppressed emotional experiencing and repression of negative affective states (Younger *et al.*, 2006). It is believed that a stress-driven activation of the opioid system would have adaptational value through blunting the potentially deleterious effect of aversive stimuli, hence enabling the individual to deal more effectively with adverse situations (Bandura *et al.*, 1988). From a neurobiological point of view, it has been recently found that the activation of opioid receptors within limbic system structures leads to a marked decrease of blood flow within the same areas (Liberzon *et al.*, 2002). One recent study has provided compelling evidence that the endogenous opioid system plays an inhibitory role in the acquisition of fear in humans (Eippert *et al.*, 2008). Using a classical fear conditioning paradigm, the researchers found that the administration of naloxone before and during the experiment enhanced the acquisition of fear, and impaired the development of habituation. These effects seemed to be caused by a mechanism which lowered threat-related activation thresholds in the amygdala.

In addition to stress-driven activation of the opioid system, there is also evidence that chronic conditions such as depression and anxiety disorders may involve a dysregulation in the opioid system (Kennedy *et al.*, 2006; Eriksson *et al.*, 1989). For example, it has been found that patients with panic disorder have abnormally high levels of endogenous opioids in cerebrospinal fluid (Eriksson *et al.*, 1989), and that their concentration increases after the induction of a panic attack with lactate (Dager *et al.*, 1989). This panic-induced release of endogenous opioids is potentially relevant to depersonalization, given that the latter is itself a prominent and frequent symptom of panic attacks (Ball *et al.*, 1997). Moreover, recent findings suggest that the experience of panic is indeed a mediating mechanism capable of triggering dissociative responses during acute trauma (Bryant and Panasetis, 2005; Nixon and Bryant, 2003). Could it be that panic-induced opioid activation may, in some circumstances, elicit depersonalization symptoms? Interestingly enough, it has been found that exposure to selective κ receptor opioid agonists reliably elicits depersonalization-derealization symptoms and dysphoria in a dose dependent manner under placebo-controlled conditions (Pfeiffer *et al.*, 1986; Walsh *et al.*, 2001).

Effect of opioid antagonists on dissociative and depersonalization symptoms

One of the interesting properties of opioid receptor antagonists is that, in the absence of concurrent opioid system activation (e.g. opiate administration or stress), they produce few discernible effects on healthy volunteers (Gutstein and Akil, 2006). As a corollary, the occurrence of marked behavioural effects following the administration of opioid antagonists may constitute an indirect sign, which suggests underlying opioid activation. In this respect, it is intriguing that opioid antagonists have been found to improve a range of 'dissociative' symptoms in patients from different diagnostic groups. For example, in order to test the hypothesis that emotional numbing is an opiate-mediated phenomenon, researchers administered nalmefene to 18 patients with post-traumatic stress disorder (PTSD), and found that eight showed a marked improvement of this and other dissociative symptoms (Glover, 1993). A similar, albeit less dramatic reduction of dissociative symptoms was observed in eight post-traumatic disorder patients (PTSD) treated with naltrexone (Lubin *et al.*, 2002). Another study tested the beneficial effect of naltrexone on 18 patients with borderline personality disorder (BPD), and found a marked reduction in both the intensity and duration of dissociative symptoms including depersonalization, emotional numbing and flashbacks (Bohus *et al.*, 1999). Although the authors did not control for placebo effects, the fact that improvements took a few days to become apparent was interpreted as suggestive of a genuine rather than placebo effect. Other researchers carried out a placebo-controlled, double-blind cross-over study to test the effects of a single dose of intravenous naloxone (0.4 mg) on nine BPD patients, whilst in an acute dissociative state. Although most patients showed significant improvement, there were no significant differences between naloxone and placebo (Philipsen *et al.*, 2004).

An interesting feature of depersonalization, which may be indicative of an overactive opioid system, is the finding of an increased pain detection threshold in patients with chronic depersonalization (Moroz *et al.*, 1990; Abugova, 1996), as well as in subjects with hypnotically induced depersonalization (Röder *et al.*, 2007). Given that the endogenous opioid system can cause suppression of both emotional and physiological pain in stress-related situations (Frew and Drummond, 2007), it is tempting to speculate that it could mediate such symptoms in depersonalization. In this regard, Russian researchers tested the hypothesis that long-lasting depersonalization stems from a dysregulation in the opioid system (Nuller *et al.*, 2001). They carried out a single-blind, placebo-controlled trial with naloxone on 14 patients suffering with long-lasting depersonalization of 1 to 16 years' duration. Six of their patients met DSM-IV criteria for depersonalization disorder with no comorbid conditions, while, in eight patients depersonalization existed concomitantly with depression. Naloxone was administered intravenously as a single dose of 1.6–4 mg in 11 patients. Three patients who failed to show any initial response were administered subsequent doses up to a maximum of 10 mg. Remarkably, the authors reported that three patients had a complete and lasting remission of depersonalization, while seven experienced significant improvement (>50% symptom reduction on a depersonalization scale). Only one patient showed moderate improvement, while in two it was minimal and short-lasting. Altogether, only one patient failed to experience any kind of symptom amelioration. In summary, 71% of their patients experienced a significant reduction in the intensity of depersonalization. Surprisingly, in most cases, symptom improvement was reported to occur within the first 20–40 min following naloxone administration. In keeping with the hypothesis that depersonalization represents an opioid-driven suppressive effect on the stress response, patients were found to have low basal plasma cortisol levels, which subsequently increased after naloxone administration.

In an attempt to further test the opioid depersonalization-model Simeon and Knutelska (2005) carried out an open-label trial with naltrexone on 14 subjects with DPD. Whilst seven subjects received a maximum dose of 100 mg/day for 6 weeks, the other seven went on to receive 250 mg/day for 10 weeks. It was found that three patients reported a marked improvement, with a more than 70% reduction in symptoms. The mean intensity reduction for the whole sample was 30% (as measured by three dissociation scales). Although these results are far less dramatic than those reported by the Russian study (Nuller *et al.*, 2001), it is worth bearing in mind that naloxone and naltrexone have different pharmacokinetic profiles, which could have an effect on results. Thus, whilst naltrexone is twice as potent as naloxone and has a considerably longer half-life, its bioavailability is more unreliable, given that it undergoes a significant first-pass effect and only 5%–12% of a dose reaches the systemic circulation (Gutstein and Akil, 2006). It is clear that more research is needed in this promising area (Simeon and Abugel, 2006).

In keeping with views of depersonalization as a stress-related inhibitory response, it is worth noticing that those neurotransmitter systems found of relevance to the condition all seem to play important inhibitory functions on the regulation of the stress response. Thus, in addition to the increasingly well-known stress-related modulatory effect of the opioid (Frew and Drummond, 2007) and serotonergic systems (Hood *et al.*, 2006), recent research has identified a glutamate-dependent fronto-limbic inhibitory mechanism on emotional behaviour (Akirav and Maroun, 2007). Indeed, glutamatergic neurons originating in the medial prefrontal cortex are thought to inhibit emotional responses, through NMDA dependent activation of inhibitory GABAergic neurons in the amygdala.

It is clear that pharmacological research on depersonalization is still in its infancy, and some of the drugs showing promising results in open-label trials need to be tested under placebo-controlled conditions in larger samples of patients. A related and needed research endeavour is to clarify the existence of clinical subgroups of depersonalization, which may show preferential response to some medications. As reviewed above, it may be that cases with a prominent background of anxiety or obsessions may respond better to SSRIs or to clonazepam. Likewise, unpublished anecdotal observations suggest that a subgroup of patients who complain of prominent attentional symptoms, underarousal and hypersomnia may respond to stimulants such as modafinil (Ballon and Feifel, 2006).

In regards to the search for new pharmacological treatments, two new drugs loom on the horizon as potentially useful: (1) cannabis receptor antagonists; (2) selective kappa opioid receptor antagonists. Indeed, given the fact that cannabis can induce depersonalization in a dose-dependent manner it would make the cannabinoid CB1 receptor antagonist rimonabant an intriguing research candidate with potential antidepersonalization effects. In line with other depersonalization-relevant neurotransmitters, the endocannabinoid system is currently thought to have a role in the modulation of emotional processes, and particularly in the mediation of adaptive responses to unavoidable stressful stimuli (Akirav and Maroun, 2007). Current research in rodents has shown rimonabant to have anxiolytic properties and to improve the deleterious effects produced by chronic stress (Griebel et al., 2005).

In view of the promising results with opioid antagonists, it is worth bearing in mind that, while the induction of depersonalization is exclusive to kappa agonists, all of the antagonists tested so far are non-specific and with a preference for mu receptors at low doses. Although kappa opioid antagonists have not yet been developed for human use, it is likely they will become available in the next few years (Metcalf and Coop, 2005).

Adapted from *Expert Rev. Neurother.* **8** (1), 19–26 (2008) with permission from Expert Reviews Ltd.

REFERENCES

Abel, K. M., Allin, M. P., Kucharska-Pietura, K. et al. (2003). Ketamine alters neural processing of facial emotion recognition in healthy men: an fMRI study. *Neuroreport*, **14**, 387–391.

Abugova, M. A. (1996). Indices of pain threshold as a method of objective assessment of depersonalization therapy efficacy. *Bekhterev Reviews in Psychiatry and Medical Psychology*, **4**, 120–122.

Akirav, I., Maroun, M. (2007).The role of the medial prefrontal cortex–amygdala circuit in stress effects on the extinction of fear. *Neural Plasticity*, **30873**. Epub Jan 16.

Anand, A., Charney, D. S., Oren, D. A. et al. (2000). Attenuation of the neuropsychiatric effects of ketamine with lamotrigine: support for hyperglutamatergic effects of N-methyl-D-aspartate receptor antagonists. *Archives of General Psychiatry*, **57**, 270–276.

Baker, D., Hunter, E., Lawrence, E. *et al.* (2003). Depersonalisation disorder: clinical features of 204 cases. *British Journal of Psychiatry*, **182**, 428–433.

Ball, S., Robinson, A., Shekhar, A., Walsh, K. (1997). Dissociative symptoms in panic disorder. *Journal of Nervous and Mental Disease*, **185**, 755–760.

Ballon, J. S., Feifel, D. (2006). A systematic review of modafinil: potential clinical uses and mechanisms of action. *The Journal of Clinical Psychiatry*, **67**, 554–566.

Bandura, A., Cioffi, D., Taylor, C.B, Brouillard, M. E. (1988). Perceived self-efficacy in coping with cognitive stressors and opioid activation. *Journal of Personality and Social Psychology*, **55**, 479–488.

Bohus, M. J., Landwehrmeyer, G. B., Stiglmayr, C. E., Limberger, M. F., Böhme, R., Schmahl, C. G. (1999). Naltrexone in the treatment of dissociative symptoms in patients with borderline personality disorder: an open-label trial. *The Journal of Clinical Psychiatry*, **60**, 598–603.

Bryant, R. A., Panasetis, P. (2005). The role of panic in acute dissociative reactions following trauma. *British Journal of Clinical Psychology*, **44**, 489–494.

Cohen, M. R., Pickar, D., Dubois, M. (1983). The role of the endogenous opioid system in the human stress response. *The Psychiatric Clinics of North America*, **6**, 457–471.

Chambers, R. A., Bremner, J. D., Moghaddam, B., Southwick, S. M., Charney, D. S., Krystal, J. H. (1999). Glutamate and post-traumatic stress disorder: toward a psychobiology of dissociation. *Seminars in Clinical Neuropsychiatry*, **4**, 274–281.

Dager, S. R., Cowley, D. S., Dorsa, D. M., Dunner, D. L. (1989). Plasma beta-endorphin response to lactate infusion. *Biological Psychiatry*, **25**, 243–245.

Davidson, J. R., Woodbury, M. A., Zisook, S., Giller, E. R. Jr. (1989). Classification of depression by grade of membership: a confirmation study. *Psychological Medicine*, **19**, 987–998.

Eippert, F., Bingel, U., Schoell, E., Yacubian, J., Büchel, C. (2008). Blockade of endogenous opioid neurotransmission enhances acquisition of conditioned fear in humans. *Journal of Neuroscience*, **28**, 5465–5472.

Eriksson, E., Westberg, P., Thuresson, K., Modigh, K., Ekman, R., Widerlöv, E. (1989). Increased cerebrospinal fluid of endorphin immunoreactivity in panic disorder. *Neuropsychopharmacology*, **2**, 225–228.

Frew, A. K., Drummond, P. D. (2007). Negative affect, pain and sex: the role of endogenous opioids. *Pain*. **132**, Suppl. 1, 577–85.

Glover, H. (1993). A preliminary trial of nalmefene for the treatment of emotional numbing in combat veterans with post-traumatic stress disorder. *The Israel Journal of Psychiatry and Related Science*, **30**, 255–263.

Goodman, and Gilman, (2001). *The Pharmacological Basis of Therapeutics*, 10th edn. New York: McGraw Hill.

Griebel, G., Stemmelin, J., Scatton, B. (2005). Effects of the cannabinoid CB1 receptor antagonist rimonabant in models of emotional reactivity in rodents. *Biological Psychiatry*, **57**, 261–267.

Gutstein, H. B., Akil, H. (2006). Opioid analgesics. In Brunton, L. L., Lazo, J. S., Parker, K. L. (eds.) *Goodman and Gilman's The Pharmacological Basis of Therapeutics*, 11th edn. New York: McGraw-Hill, pp. 577–578.

Hill, M. N., Sun, J. C., Tse, M. T., Gorzalka, B. B. (2006). Altered responsiveness of serotonin receptor subtypes following long-term cannabinoid treatment. *The International Journal of Neuropsychopharmacology*, **9**, 277–286.

Hollander, E., Liebowitz, M. R., DeCaria, C., Fairbanks, J., Fallon, B., Klein, D. F. (1990). Treatment of depersonalization with serotonin reuptake blockers. *The Journal of Clinical Psychopharmacology*, **10**, 200–203.

Hood, S. D., Hince, D. A., Robinson, H. (2006). Serotonin regulation of the human stress response. *Psychoneuroendocrinology*, **31**, 1087–1097.

Kennedy, S. E., Koeppe, R. A., Young, E. A., Zubieta, J.K. (2006). Dysregulation of endogenous opioid emotion regulation circuitry in major depression in women. *Archives of General Psychiatry*, **63**, 1199–1208.

Krystal, J. H., Karper, L. P., Seibyl, J. P. *et al.* (1994). Subanesthetic effects of the non-competitive NMDA antagonist, ketamine, in humans. Psychotomimetic, perceptual, cognitive, and neuroendocrine responses. *Archives of General Psychiatry*, **51**, 199–214.

Lambert, M. V., Senior, C., Phillips, M. L., David, A. S. (2000). Depersonalization in cyberspace. *Journal of Nervous and Mental Disease*, **188**, 764–771.

Liberzon, I., Zubieta, J. K., Fig, L. M., Phan, K. L., Koeppe, R. A., Taylor, S. F. (2002). Mu-opioid receptors and limbic responses to aversive emotional stimuli. *Proceedings of the National Academy of Sciences*, USA, **99**, 7084–7089.

Lubin, G., Weizman, A., Shmushkevitz, M., Valevski, A. (2002). Short-term treatment of post-traumatic stress disorder with naltrexone: an open-label preliminary study. *Human Psychopharmacology*, **17**, 181–185.

Mathew, R. J., Wilson, W. H., Humphreys, D., Lowe, J. V., Weithe, K. E. (1993). Depersonalization after marijuana smoking. *Biological Psychiatry*, **33**, 431–441.

Melges, F. T., Tinklenberg, J. R., Hollister, L. E., Gillespie, H. K. (1970). Temporal disintegration and depersonalization during marihuana intoxication. *Archives of General Psychiatry*, **23**, 204–210.

Metcalf, M. D., Coop, A. (2005). Kappa opioid antagonists: past successes and future prospects. *AAPS Journal*, **7**, 704–722.

Moroz, B. T., Nuller, I. L., Ustimova, I. N., Andreev, B. V. (1990). Study of pain sensitivity based on the indicators of electro-odontometry in patients with depersonalization and depressive disorders. *Zhurnal Nevropatologii Psikhiatrii Imeni S S Korsakova*, **90**, 81–82.

Nakazi, M., Bauer, U., Nickel, T., Kathmann, M., Schlicker, E. (2000). Inhibition of serotonin release in the mouse brain via presynaptic cannabinoid CB1 receptors. *Naunyn-Schmiedeberg's Archives of Pharmacology*, **361**, 19–24.

Nixon, R. D., Bryant, R. A. (2003). Peritraumatic and persistent panic attacks in acute stress disorder. *Behavior Research Therapy*, **41**, 1237–1242.

Nuller, Y. L. (1982). Depersonalisation – symptoms, meaning, therapy. *Acta Psychiatrica Scandinavica*, **66**, 451–458.

Nuller, Y. L., Morozova, M. G., Kushnir, O. N., Hamper, N. (2001). Effect of naloxone therapy on depersonalization: a pilot study. *Journal of Psychopharmacology*, **15**, 93–95.

Pfeiffer, A., Brantl, V., Herz, A., Emrich, H. M. (1986). Psychotomimesis mediated by kappa opiate receptors. *Science*, **233**, 774–776.

Philipsen, A., Schmahl, C., Lieb, K. (2004). Naloxone in the treatment of acute dissociative states in female patients with borderline personality disorder. *Pharmacopsychiatry*, **37**, 196–199.

Phillips, M. L., Medford, N., Senior, C. *et al.* (2001). Depersonalization disorder: thinking without feeling. *Psychiatry Research: Neuroimaging*, **108**, 145–160.

Resnick, O., Krus, D. M., Raskin, M. (1964). LSD-25 in normal subjects treated with monoamine oxidase inhibitor. *Life Sciences*, **3**, 1207–1214.

Röder, C. H., Michal, M., Overbeck, G., van de Ven, V. G., Linden, D. E. (2007). Pain response in depersonalization: a functional imaging study using hypnosis in healthy subjects. *Psychotherapy and Psychosomatics*, **76**, 115–121.

Russo, E. B., Burnett, A., Hall, B., Parker, K. K. (2005). Agonistic properties of cannabidiol at 5-HT1a receptors. *Neurochemical Research*, **30**, 1037–1043.

Sachdev, P. (2002). Citalopram–clonazepam combination for primary depersonalization disorder: a case report. The *Australian and New Zealand Journal of Psychiatry*, **36**, 424–425.

Sedman, G., Kenna, J. C. (1964). The occurrence of depersonalization phenomena under LSD. *Psychiatria et Neurologia (Basel)*, **147**, 129–137.

Sierra, M., Phillips, M. L., Lambert, M. V., Senior, C., David, A. S., Krystal, J. H. (2001). Lamotrigine in the treatment of depersonalization disorder. *The Journal of Clinical Psychiatry*, **62**, 826–827.

Sierra, M., Phillips, M. L., Ivin, G., Krystal, J., David, A. S. (2003). A placebo-controlled, cross-over trial of lamotrigine in depersonalization disorder. *Journal of Psychopharmacology*, **17**, 103–105.

Sierra, M., Baker, D., Medford, N., Lawrence, E., Patel, M., Phillips, M. L., David, A. S. (2006). Lamotrigine as an add-on treatment for depersonalization disorder: a retrospective study of 32 cases. *Clinical Neuropharmacology*, **29**, 253–839.

Simeon, D., Abugel, J. (2006). *Feeling Unreal: Depersonalization Disorder and the Loss of Self*. Oxford: Oxford University Press.

Simeon, D., Knutelska, M. (2005). An open trial of naltrexone in the treatment of depersonalization disorder. *Clinical Journal of Psychopharmacology*, **25**, 267–270.

Simeon, D., Hollander, E., Stein, D. J. *et al.* (1995). Induction of depersonalization by the serotonin agonist meta-chlorophenylpiperazine. *Psychiatry Research*, **58**, 161–164.

Simeon, D., Stein, D. J., Hollander, E. (1998). Treatment of depersonalization disorder with clomipramine. *Biological Psychiatry*, **44**, 302–303.

Simeon, D., Knutelska, M., Nelson, D., Guralnik, O. (2003). Feeling unreal: a depersonalization disorder update of 117 cases. *The Journal of Clinical Psychiatry*, **64**, 990–997.

Simeon, D., Guralnik, O., Schmeidler, J., Knutelska, M. (2004). Fluoxetine therapy in depersonalisation disorder: randomised controlled trial. *The British Journal of Psychiatry*, **185**, 31–36.

Stein, M. B., Uhde, T. W. (1989). Depersonalization disorder: effects of caffeine and response to pharmacotherapy. *Biological Psychiatry*, **26**, 315–320.

Wittmann, M., Carter, O., Hasler, F. *et al.* (2007). Effects of psilocybin on time perception and temporal control of behaviour in humans. *Journal of Psychopharmacology*, **21**, 50–64.

Younger, J. W., Lawler-Row, K. A., Moe, K. A., Kratz, A. L., Keenum, A. J. (2006). Effects of naltrexone on repressive coping and disclosure of emotional material: a test of the opioid–peptide hypothesis of repression and hypertension. *Psychosomatic Medicine*, **68**, 734–741.

Walsh, S. L., Strain, E. C., Abreu, M. E., Bigelow, G. E. (2001). Enadoline, a selective kappa opioid agonist: comparison with butorphanol and hydromorphone in humans. *Psychopharmacology (Berlin)*, **157**, 151–162.

9

Psychological approaches to the treatment of depersonalization disorder

Introduction

Most published reports on psychological treatments for depersonalization have been mainly anecdotal or confined to small series of cases (Hunter *et al.*, 2003). Such reports mention a whole range of approaches, including behavioural (Sookman and Solyom, 1978; Dollinger, 1983), as well as psychoanalytical (Torch, 1987). Unfortunately, the lack of quantified, systematic studies makes it difficult to assess the value of the approaches used. Nevertheless, beneficial psychological approaches to depersonalization seem to be informed by one of three different conceptual frameworks which emphasize different aspects of the condition. In what follows, the main features of each of these approaches will be considered.

Psychodynamic therapy

Early authors writing on the usefulness of orthodox psychoanalytical approaches to depersonalization concurred on the view that successful outcomes were difficult to achieve, and were said to take on average twice as long as treatment for other neurotic conditions. Some indeed advocated no less than 5 years of intensive psychotherapy (Schilder, 1939). More recent authors have taken a less pessimistic attitude and have reported the use of psychodynamic-informed psychotherapy to be useful in some patients with depersonalization disorder (Torch, 1987). In such an approach, 'fear of losing control' has been emphasized as a central therapeutic target. Indeed, as discussed in Chapter 7, it is likely that an extreme sensitivity to 'control' threats plays an important role in psychological mechanisms that trigger and maintain depersonalization. Such vulnerability is thought to arise from developmental difficulties in the establishment of a healthy 'narcissism' and a trusting relationship with significant others (Michal *et al.*, 2006). In this regard, it is not surprising that a significant correlation has been found between depersonalization in adulthood and experiences of emotional abuse during childhood (Simeon *et al.*, 2001; Michal *et al.*, 2007). Such 'abuse' or neglect can often be subtle and implicit in certain life events rather than purposely perpetrated. For example, a number of adverse life events during childhood seem over-represented in patients with depersonalization disorder. For example, divorce of parents during childhood; having had cold and distant parents; having been sent to a boarding school at an early age; having been placed in adult-like roles of responsibility, such as caring for an ailing relative, or having been subjected to significant bullying at school without adequate protection from significant adults. Other patients, in whom such a history is not present, typically are only children or gifted individuals coming from families where achievement is over-emphasized and where parents relate to them as objects for their own narcissistic gratification, rather than as whole beings (Torch, 1987). Schilder (1951), who was clearly aware of these childhood antecedents, stated: "I am inclined to stress the fact that the patient with depersonalization has been admired very much by the parents for his intellectual and physical gifts ... The final outcome of such an attitude by the parents will not be different from the outcome of an attitude of neglect" (p. 276). Indeed, a likely developmental outcome of both kinds of rearing backgrounds is that individuals become overtly dependent on external sources of approval to construe and sustain a sense of self (Torch, 1987). It has been proposed that, as such relational needs become internalized into self-structure, the individual begins to privilege a sense of self as a performing object ('third person viewpoint'), rather than as a source of subjective experiencing ('first person viewpoint'). Such a deep-seated identification with an object-like view of the self manifests itself as pervasive self-observation, coupled with an actual negation of subjective experiencing: "...by identification with the parents, self-observation will take the place of the observation by others" (Schilder, 1951, p. 276). Such a state of affairs places a tremendous emphasis on a need to live up to standards imposed by a tyrannical and unrealistically idealized self (which is, in turn, an indirect reflection of perceived impositions by significant others). It goes without saying that patients with depersonalization disorder often find themselves trapped in a lost battle, which ensures a constant sense of inadequacy and feelings of lack of control. The latter, in turn, are likely to trigger and sustain feelings of depersonalization. In this regard, the condition has been characterized as a disorder of the narcissistic regulation of self-esteem (Michal *et al.*, 2006). However, as discussed by Mann and Havens (1987) "the vulnerability to depersonalized states, we suggest, lies not in the *level* of self esteem, but in its *genuineness*. One fails to own the impulses and ideas that are truly one's own. At the same time, the reflective self that should do the owning is somehow left out of the picture" (p. 148). A recent study has marshalled empirical evidence that provides some validation to the above psychodynamic views. The research compared 35 patients with pathological depersonalization with 28 patient controls along validated measures of narcissistic self-regulation (German Narcissism Inventory) and interpersonal behaviour (Inventory of Interpersonal Problems). It was found that patients with depersonalization were characterized by more pronounced 'subjectively experienced threat' and a negative view of others. Additionally, they perceived themselves as socially alienated, exceedingly helpless, hopeless, and worthless (Michal *et al.*, 2006). The authors suggest that such subjective experiences might generate a self-perpetuating cycle, whereby experienced emotional abuse during childhood leads to feelings of alienation and inadequacy (e.g. shame), which in turn, lead to avoidance of social contact, withdrawal from reality and detachment from their own self. Depersonalization itself then becomes a source of further inadequacy feelings, shame and alienation, generating, in turn, more depersonalization and so forth (Michal *et al.*, 2006).

Although the effectiveness of insight-orientated psychotherapy on depersonalization has not been systematically assessed, single case reports suggest that it can be beneficial in selected patients. A desirable goal of therapy should be for the patient to realize that depersonalization and associated feelings of worthlessness and helplessness stem from unrealistic parental expectations, and their subsequent introjection into a tyrannical idealized self, whose demands can never be met.

Abreaction: the release of suppressed emotions

Abreaction, the emotional reliving of traumatic events, usually facilitated by hypnosis, or central nervous system depressants such as barbiturates and benzodiazepines, can be a useful therapeutic intervention in the treatment of victims of trauma. Although first described by Bleuler and Freud in the treatment of hysterical symptoms, it was only during the two World Wars that abreaction was systematically used on patients with psychiatric conditions. One of the pioneers in the use of abreaction on victims of war was the British psychiatrist, Hyam J. Shorvon, who also happened to have an interest in cases of chronic depersonalization not related to any obvious traumatic situations. In his paper 'the depersonalization syndrome', Shorvon (1946) described a number of treatments such as electroconvulsive therapy (ECT), vasodilators, etc., which were tried with very little or no benefit. An intriguing exception, however, was the use of ether-induced abreaction, which was tried on 14 patients with chronic depersonalization. It was found that four cases showed a dramatic remission after one single abreaction session, while seven showed variable degrees of improvement. Overall, only three cases failed to show any improvement after abreaction; a surprising finding in view of the non-traumatic origin of most cases. Indeed, it was found that a triggering traumatic event was not required for the treatment to be effective: "successful abreaction can be carried out around non-specific incidents whose only use is that they can release a sufficient degree of excitement" (Shorvon and Sargent, 1947, p. 719). The authors endorsed a Pavlovian model according to which certain neurotic symptoms arose as a consequence of abnormal, tonic inhibitions on areas of the cerebral cortex (Sargent and Shorvon, 1945): "when there is a useful response to abreaction there are generally hysterical or reactive depressive components to the total picture, or an accompanying state of depersonalization. All these suggest the presence of inhibitory phenomena which excitation under ether may loosen" (Shorvon and Sargent, 1947, p. 725).

A more recent report of the use of abreaction in depersonalization was the case of a 55-year-old woman with a 35-year history of chronic, primary depersonalization, and a number of failed trials with antidepressants, antipsychotics and stimulants as well as ECT (Ballard *et al.*, 1992). During the course of a brief, psychoanalytically orientated therapy, it became clear that she harboured anger and destructive feelings towards her mother. It seemed, however, that the attainment of that insight made no difference to her depersonalization symptoms. She then underwent a session of abreactive therapy: "After intravenously receiving 10 mg of diazepam in 20 ml water she initially appeared relaxed, but suddenly became angry and hostile when her mother was introduced into the conversation. She vehemently protested her hatred for her mother and expressed a wish for her mother to die. This phase lasted about 2 to 3 minutes before she started becoming drowsy and eventually fell asleep" (Ballard *et al.*, 1992, p. 124). During the following session the patient reported feeling anxious and panicky but claimed not to feel depersonalized any more. Subsequent follow-up sessions showed the remission of depersonalization to be stable, and her residual anxiety was successfully treated with anxiety management techniques. In view of the promising results reported from the use of abreactive techniques, it is surprising that no further studies have been carried out. Although rarely used as originally described, abreactive techniques are still in use, not only to aid the recovery and integration of dissociated traumatic material, but also in the reintegration of emotions when they have become dissociated from thoughts of perceptions as is the case of depersonalization. Currently, hypnosis is the method of choice to facilitate abreaction, and a range of techniques have been described for its induction and management (Putnam, 1992).

Although there are no recent systematic studies on the use of abreactive techniques on patients with depersonalization disorder, in the author's experience the use of imagery-driven techniques (Smucker *et al.*, 1995; Holmer *et al.*, 2007) can allow managed, therapeutic abreaction in depersonalization disorder patients with a history of emotional abuse. Such abreactive experiences can produce a lasting amelioration of symptoms in some patients. In those with severe emotional numbing, the use of hypnotic regression to a time before the onset of symptoms can sometimes allow patients to transiently re-experience emotional feelings. Such instances can act as a powerful experiential challenge to strong held assumptions about the irreversibility of emotional numbing, and can catalyse further therapeutic gains. To conclude, sporadic, anecdotal observations suggest that the use of abreactive techniques may have a promising role in the treatment of depersonalization. It is clear that this is an area in need of much systematic research.

Cognitive-behavioural therapy

A recent cognitive-behavioural model of depersonalization disorder (Hunter *et al.*, 2003) proposes that the condition may result from catastrophic misinterpretations of normally occurring and fleeting depersonalization symptoms. It is indeed common for patients to frequently interpret depersonalization symptoms as impending signs of madness, neurological illness or irreversible brain damage caused by drugs (Baker *et al.*, 2003; 2007b). These misinterpretations become threatening in themselves, exacerbate anxiety and no-control-feelings, which in turn can elicit more depersonalization, hence perpetuating it in a self-sustaining cycle (Hunter *et al.*, 2003). The distressing nature of depersonalization also frequently leads patients to start avoiding those situations that increase the intensity of symptoms (e.g. social situations). As is the case with phobic behaviours in general, such avoidance only serves to perpetuate the very anxiety and lack of control feelings that are likely to trigger and sustain depersonalization.

Based on this cognitive-behavioural model Hunter *et al.* (2003) have outlined a number of interventions, which have been found beneficial in a recent open-label trial on 21 patients with depersonalization disorder (Hunter *et al.*, 2005). The following are the main therapeutic principles advocated by these authors; for a detailed description of such techniques and interventions, see Baker *et al.* (2007a).

Psycho-education and normalizing

Given the role of wrong assumptions regarding the nature of depersonalization, it is to be expected that adequate knowledge and understanding of the condition should result in an attenuation of the catastrophic interpretations deemed to be important in the maintenance of depersonalization symptoms. The importance of psychoeducation is underlined by the fact that patients have been frequently suffering with the condition for years, and have usually received no small amount of conflicting information. It has been found, in fact, that the average elapsed time until the condition gets to be diagnosed is 7–12 years (Hunter *et al.*, 2003). A common scenario is that of symptoms being disregarded, misdiagnosed or treated as irrelevant manifestations of other conditions such as anxiety, depression or even impending psychosis. Needless to say, such predicament generates significant amounts of confusion, distress, anger and feelings of helplessness and hopelessness. Not surprisingly, patients experience an extraordinary relief when they realize that their often bewildering array of symptoms is the manifestation of a well-defined syndrome. Moreover, presenting depersonalization as a fairly common protective psychological distancing mechanism, which on occasions can become chronic, offers a cognitive re-framing which has a normalizing and empowering effect.

Diary keeping

In keeping with its established role in cognitive-behavioural therapy (CBT), diary keeping has been found useful to highlight to patients the extent to which their symptoms change from moment to moment. This may come as a surprise to patients who are adamant that their symptoms do not fluctuate in intensity. Diary keeping can also be useful in helping patients identify possible predictable patterns and the effects that different activities or states of mind have on the intensity of the symptoms. Such information can be used in turn to implement behavioural prescriptions intended to prevent avoidance behaviour, and to foster activities which bring about symptom amelioration (Hunter et al., 2003, 2005).

Avoidance reduction

Typical situations avoided by depersonalization sufferers are those usually resulting in increased anxiety and depersonalization, such as social situations, crowded public places and driving (Hunter et al., 2003). In this regard, managed exposure to avoided situations, as well as the implementation of other techniques such as the use of role playing, relevant to social situations, has been found to be useful (Sookman and Solyom, 1978; Hunter et al., 2005).

Reduction of self-focused attention

'Refocusing' and 'grounding techniques' which direct attention to predetermined objects, images or self-statements have been advocated in the treatment of depersonalization, as they may help to interrupt the constant symptom monitoring in which many patients engage (Hunter et al., 2003, 2005).

Challenging catastrophic assumptions

As mentioned above, catastrophic assumptions are thought to play a central role in the maintenance of depersonalization. It is therefore important to ask patients about their fears regarding the meaning of depersonalization. These catastrophic interpretations can then be gradually challenged, initially by means of psychoeducation, and later on, once the therapeutic alliance has been well established, by means of experimentation and evidence gathering (Hunter et al., 2003; Baker et al., 2007a).

In the CBT open trial mentioned above, the authors found significant improvements on self-rated measures of depersonalization, as well as anxiety, depression and general functioning. In fact, it was found that 29% of participants no longer met criteria for depersonalization disorder at the end of therapy. A follow-up 6 months later showed the latter gains to be stable. These initial results strongly suggest that a CBT approach to depersonalization may be effective at least for a subgroup of patients. However, given that there was no control group, it is difficult to ascertain a specific role of the techniques used. Be it as it may, however, an important general conclusion to be derived from the evidence reviewed in this chapter is that, far from being the unassailable rock early writers led us to believe, depersonalization disorder has been shown to be amenable to psychological interventions.

Although stemming from different theoretical frameworks and sets of observations, the three models discussed in this chapter are not necessarily mutually incompatible and principles deriving from all three could be used in selected cases, as they inform different aspects of the condition. Thus, the psychodynamic approach emphasizes triggering and sustaining mechanisms centred on lack of control feelings and perceived threat to self. Abreactive techniques, in turn, may provide a yet to be further explored strategy to deal with the more dissociative aspects of the condition. Lastly, CBT is likely to deal better with the more cognitive, anxiety-generating mechanisms, which sustain the condition and constitute a major source of distress and incapacity.

REFERENCES

Baker, D., Hunter, E., Lawrence, E., David, A. (2007a). *Overcoming Depersonalization and Feelings of Unreality: A Self-help Guide Using Cognitive Behavioural Techniques.* London: Constable and Robinson.

Baker, D., Earle, M., Medford, N., Sierra, M., Towell, A., David, A. S. (2007b). Illness perceptions in depersonalization disorder: testing an illness Attribution Model. *Clinical Psychology and Psychotherapy*, **14**, 105–116.

Ballard, C. G., Mohan, R. N., Handy, S. (1992). Chronic depersonalisation neurosis au Shorvon – a successful intervention. *British Journal of Psychiatry*, **160**, 123–125.

Dollinger, S. J. (1983). A case report of dissociative neurosis (depersonalization disorder) in an adolescent treated with family therapy and behavior modification. *Journal of Consulting and Clinical Psychology*, **51**, 479–484.

Holmer, E. A., Arntz, A., Smucher, M. R. (2007). Imagery rescripting in cognitive behaviour therapy: images, treatment techniques and outcomes. *Journal of Behavior Therapy and Experimental Psychiatry*, **38**, 297–305.

Hunter, E. C., Phillips, M. L., Chalder, T., Sierra, M., David, A. S. (2003). Depersonalisation disorder: a cognitive-behavioural conceptualisation. *Behaviour Research and Therapy*, **41**, 1451–1467.

Hunter, E. C., Baker, D., Phillips, M. L., Sierra, M., David, A. S. (2005). Cognitive-behaviour therapy for depersonalisation disorder: an open study. *Behaviour Research and Therapy*, **43**, 1121–1130.

Mann, D. W., Havens, L. L. (1987). Discussion of Dr Torch's paper: depersonalization and the pathology of the self. *The Hillside Journal of Clinical Psychiatry*, **9**, 144–151.

Michal, M., Kaufhold, J., Overbeck, G., Grabhorn, R. (2006). Narcissistic regulation of the self and interpersonal problems in depersonalized patients. *Psychopathology*, **39**, 192–198.

Michal, M., Beutel, M. E., Jordan, J., Zimmermann, M., Wolters, S., Heidenreich, T. (2007). Depersonalization, mindfulness, and childhood trauma. *Journal of Nervous and Mental Disease*, **195**, 693–696.

Miller, F., Bashkin, E. A. (1974). Depersonalization and self-mutilation. *Psychoanaytic Quarterly*, **43**, 638–649.

Putnam, F. W. (1992). Using hypnosis for therapeutic abreactions. *Psychiatric Medicine*, **10**, 51–65.

Sargant, W., Shorvon, H. J. (1945). Acute war neurosis. *Archives of Neurology and Psychiatry*, **54**, 231–245.

Shorvon, H. J. (1946). The depersonalisation syndrome. *Proceedings of the Royal Society of Medicine*, **39**, 779–792.

Shorvon, H. J., Sargant, W. (1947). Excitatory abreaction; with special reference to its mechanism and the use of ether. *Journal of Mental Science*, **93**, 709–732.

Simeon, D., Guralnik, O., Schmeidler, J., Sirof, B., Knutelska, M. (2001). The role of childhood interpersonal trauma in depersonalization disorder. *American Journal of Psychiatry*, **158**, 1027–1033.

Schilder, P. F. (1939). Treatment of depersonalization. *Bulletin of the New York Academy of Medicine*, **15**, 258–266.

Schilder, P. F. (1951). *Psychotherapy*. London, Routledge & Kegan Paul Ltd.

Smucker, M. R., Dancu, C. V., Foa, E. B., Niederee, J. L. (1995). Imagery rescripting: a new treatment for survivors of childhood sexual abuse suffering from posttraumatic stress. *Journal of Cognitive Psychotherapy: An International Quarterly*, **9**, 3–17.

Sookman, D., Solyom, L. (1978). Severe depersonalization treated by behavior therapy. *American Journal of Psychiatry*, **135**, 1543–1545.

Torch, E. M. (1987). The psychotherapeutic treatment of depersonalization disorder. *The Hillside Journal of Clinical Psychiatry*, **9**, 133–151.

10

The neurobiology of depersonalization

Introduction

Unlike the case with most psychopathological phenomena where subjective reports are usually associated with objective behavioural manifestations, the distressing complaints of patients with depersonalization do not seem accompanied by observable changes in behaviour. In spite of this, there is now a growing body of evidence revealing a number of neurobiological abnormalities in patients with depersonalization disorder.

Autonomic response

It was Lader and Wing (1966) who first published the intriguing, serendipitous observation of a patient in whom the onset of depersonalization during a panic-like attack was accompanied by a dramatic flattening of her previously labile galvanic skin response (GSR):

I was recording the skin resistance from an anxious female and a typical tracing with low resistance, many fluctuations and discernible GSR to external stimuli was being obtained ... Then, fairly abruptly, the skin resistance rose to high levels and became flat and unresponsive, and the pulse rate dropped. On questioning later, the patient described how she had been feeling more and more panicky and was about to cry out for help when the anxiety suddenly subsided to be replaced by a strange feeling of detachment. Sounds appeared distant, vision was blurred and 'swimmy' and the patient's limbs felt as if they did not belong to her. On three subsequent occasions with other patients I have noted similar short term changes. (Lader and Wing, 1966, p. 69).

An even earlier work, looking at the psychophysiological effects of repeated electrical shocks on healthy subjects, had reported that, at the time of receiving high intensity shocks, subjects often described feelings of derealization or of becoming detached observers of themselves. Coinciding with this, there was a blunting in their skin conductance recordings (Oswald, 1959). Incidentally, a less dramatic confirmation of such findings has recently been obtained.

Sixty-nine undergraduate students were exposed to a succession of 19 aversive auditory probes, while their skin conductance responses were measured. It was found that the occurrence of acute dissociative experiences (including depersonalization), during the experiment was associated with a fast attenuation of skin conductance responses (i.e. habituation) (Giesbrecht et al., 2008).

A study carried out in the late 1960s reported findings on the sympathetic autonomic system in patients suffering with continuous, chronic depersonalization states (Kelly and Walter, 1968). Using forearm blood flow as a measurement of sympathetic autonomic function, the authors found that a group of eight 'depersonalized patients' had the lowest 'basal' recordings, as compared with groups of patients suffering from the following conditions: chronic anxiety, non-agitated depression, agitated depression, schizophrenia, phobic states, obsessional neurosis, personality disorders, hysteria and normal controls. These findings suggested an abnormally low tone in the sympathetic autonomic nervous system. The highest basal autonomic activity was observed in the chronic anxiety group, which was almost four times higher than that observed in the depersonalization group. In contrast, however, it was found that subjective ratings of anxiety were slightly higher in the depersonalization group than in the anxiety group. Such a counterintuitive finding led the researchers to conclude: "The evidence suggests that the discrepancy between subjective and objective signs of anxiety is the fundamental characteristic of patients with depersonalization. In physiological terms, anxiety is experienced but is not translated into defence reaction arousal" (Walter and Kelly, 1968). In keeping with such findings, a study on a group of patients with anxiety disorder found that the presence of depersonalization accounted for much of the variance of electrodermal habituation rate (Rabavilas, 1989).

A more recent study tested the prediction that the observed attenuation of sympathetic autonomic responses was selective to emotional stimuli rather than a non-specific low arousal state (Sierra et al., 2002). The skin conductance responses of 15 patients with depersonalization disorder, 15 controls, and 11 individuals with anxiety disorders were recorded in response to non-specific elicitors of electrodermal responses (an unexpected clap and taking a sigh) and in response to pictures with neutral and emotional contents. The unpleasant pictures showed scary, disgusting scenes such as dismembered bodies, snakes poised to attack, accidents, etc. Pleasant pictures showed attractive animals, couples kissing, etc. whilst the neutral pictures depicted uninteresting objects such as a hair dryer, a light bulb, etc. As can be seen in Fig. 10.1, it was found that the depersonalization patients had selectively reduced autonomic responses to unpleasant pictures, but not to neutral or pleasant ones (the response to the latter was also reduced, but the difference was not statistically significant). Also, the latency of response to these stimuli was prolonged significantly in the group with depersonalization disorder. In contrast, latency to non-specific stimuli (clap and sigh) was significantly shorter in the depersonalization and anxiety groups than in the healthy controls.

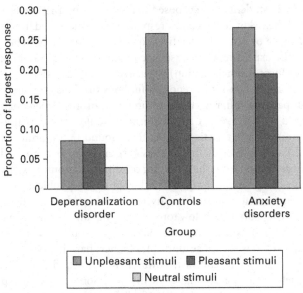

Fig. 10.1. Skin conductance response (SCR) magnitude to stimuli across groups. Because amplitudes can vary across participants, responses are standardized as range corrected scores (for each participant, SCR magnitudes were computed as a proportion of that participant's largest response) (taken from Sierra *et al.*, 2002).

These findings suggested the presence of both inhibitory and facilitatory mechanisms on autonomic arousal, which pointed to a specific disruption in emotional information processing rather than a non-specific dampening effect on autonomic reactivity.

Interestingly, in spite of their attenuated autonomic responses to the unpleasant pictures, patients with depersonalization were perfectly capable of rating the experienced unpleasantness of each picture (i.e. valence), although they rated them as less subjectively arousing.

Another related study compared the skin conductance responses of depersonalization disorder patients with those of anxiety disorder patients and normal controls, as they watched pictures and video clips of facial expressions of disgust and happiness (Sierra *et al.*, 2006). It was found that, whilst patients in the anxiety group had increased autonomic reactivity to disgust expressions, depersonalization patients had very similar responses to those of the healthy controls (see Fig. 10.2). This was surprising, given that both the depersonalization and the anxiety patients had reported similarly high levels of subjective anxiety, as measured by administered anxiety scales. In other words, in spite of acknowledging high subjective anxiety, the autonomic responses of depersonalization patients resembled those of healthy controls rather than those of

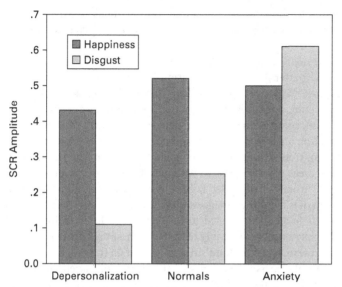

Fig. 10.2. Mean log-transformed to disgust and happy facial expressions across the three groups (from Sierra, M., Senior, C., Phillips, M. L., David, A. S., 2006).

similarly anxious patients diagnosed with anxiety disorders (anxiety disorder group). Such findings converge with those reported in earlier studies (Walter and Kelly, 1968; Sierra *et al.*, 2002), and suggest that the presence of depersonalization in otherwise anxious patients has a blunting and selective effect on autonomic reactivity. Thus, it would seem that this attenuation effect is not absolute but relative to anxiety levels. This idea finds further support in a study which compared the levels of urinary norepinephrine of patients with depersonalization disorder and healthy controls. In keeping with their higher anxiety levels, patients with depersonalization were found to have higher levels of norepinephrine than their controls. However, within the depersonalization group itself, there was a striking norepinephrine reduction with increasing levels of depersonalization (Simeon *et al.*, 2003). To conclude, it seems plausible to suggest that autonomic responses in patients with depersonalization are likely to reflect a balance between two opposing tendencies: an excitatory one determined by anxiety levels, and an inhibitory one determined by depersonalization intensity.

Functional neuroimaging studies

Over the last decade a number of studies using functional neuroimaging in depersonalization disorder patients have been published. Such studies are not only beginning to show evidence of brain dysfunctional activity, but also show how those abnormal findings relate to the autonomic changes already discussed.

One of the first neuroimaging studies used positron emission tomography (PET), to compare patterns of brain activation of eight patients with depersonalization disorder with normal controls as they performed a verbal memory task (Simeon *et al.*, 2000). Although patients showed reduced metabolic activity in some association areas such as the right superior and middle temporal gyri, other association areas in the parietal and occipital lobes, were more active than those in the controls. The finding of anomalous activation patterns in cross-modal association areas seems consistent with long-held views that depersonalization may result from a high-order failure of cortical integration (Ackner, 1954). In particular, it is tempting to suggest that the abnormal parietal activation mentioned above is functionally related to the feelings of disembodiment and anomalous body experiencing commonly reported by these patients (Sierra *et al.*, 2005). In fact, the researchers reported a striking correlation ($r = 0.7$) between the subjective intensity of depersonalization and the degree of parietal increased activation (Simeon *et al.*, 2000).

Other studies using functional neuroimaging have been designed to explore the neural underpinnings of emotional numbing in depersonalization. The first of those studies used functional magnetic resonance imaging (fMRI) to compare the neural response of patients with depersonalization disorder with that of healthy volunteers and patients with obsessive compulsive disorder. Participants were scanned as they watched a series of aversive and neutral pictures extracted from a well-known and standardized set (the international affective picture system; IAPS). Attesting to the presence of subjective emotional numbing, depersonalized patients stated that, although they could understand the content of the pictures, they failed to experience any subjective emotional response (Phillips *et al.*, 2001).

It was found that whilst healthy controls as well as OCD patients showed activation in the anterior insula in response to unpleasant and disgusting pictures, such activation was not seen in the patients with depersonalization. As will be discussed in the next chapter, the insula seems to play an important role in the process that allows feelings to become conscious (Craig, 2009). Other brain areas, also known to be relevant in the response to expressions of fear and disgust, such as the occipito-temporal cortex, were also found to be underactive in patients with depersonalization as compared with the two control groups (see Fig. 10.3).

Another key finding of this study was that depersonalization patients, but not the controls, showed an area of activation in the right ventrolateral prefrontal cortex (BA 47). This region seemed functionally coupled with the insula. Indeed, during the presentation of unpleasant pictures, there was evidence of an inverse correlation, so that prefrontal activation only occurred in the absence of

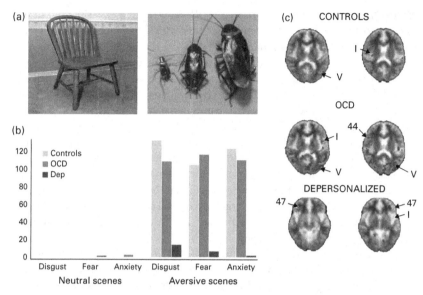

Fig. 10.3. (a) Depersonalized patients, those with obsessive compulsive disorder (OCD) and normal controls viewed alternating series of neutral and aversive scenes from a standardized series. One example each of the neutral (left) and aversive (right) scenes are depicted. (b) Median total scores for subjective ratings of neutral and aversive scenes are shown for all three-subject groups on three dimensions: disgust, fear and anxiety. (c) Two transverse brain slices from brain activation maps acquired with fMRI representing group-averaged neuronal activity to aversive (dark grey) and neutral scenes (light grey) are shown for all three groups. The left side of the brain is on the right side of the image, and vice versa. In normal controls major regions of neuronal activity in response to aversive scenes are shown in the right insula (I), and visual cortex (V). In OCD patients major regions of neuronal activity in response to aversive scenes are shown in the left insula (I); visual cortex (V), and right dorsolateral prefrontal frontal cortex (Brodmann Area 44). Neither group demonstrated significant neuronal activity in response to the neutral scenes. In depersonalized patients major regions of neuronal activity are shown primarily in response to the neutral scenes in the left insula (I) and left ventrolateral prefrontal cortex (Brodmann Area 47), and in response to the aversive scenes in right ventrolateral prefrontal frontal cortex (Brodmann Area 47) (from Phillips *et al.*, 2001).

insula activation. Interestingly, the prefrontal area in question (Brodmann Area 47) has been implicated in the evaluation of negative or aversive information, and on exerting control over both emotional experience and its impact on decision-making. For example, activation of this and other related frontal regions has been observed when normal subjects attempt to control emotional responses to negative pictures by viewing the picture with a sense of detachment or by imagining a positive unfolding of the depicted scenario (Beer *et al.*,

2006; Quirk *et al.*, 2006). In a related fMRI study, with a experimental design similar to the one described above patients with depersonalization disorder were scanned when symptomatic, and following remission of symptoms after successful treatment (Medford, 2006; and personal communication). In short, 14 patients experiencing constant depersonalization were initially scanned and found to have a pattern of activation very similar to that reported by Phillips *et al.*, 2002 in response to unpleasant emotional pictures: activation of the right ventrolateral prefrontal cortex (BA47), and lack of activation in insula and amygdala in response to unpleasant emotional pictures. After approximately 6 months of pharmacological treatment, five patients were found to have had significant clinical improvement, while the other five had been unresponsive to treatment. Findings at follow-up revealed that those in the 'responder' group no longer showed activation of the right prefrontal cortex (BA47) in response to aversive pictures and revealed significant left insula activation as compared with the 'non-responder' group.

Another recent fMRI study has marshalled further evidence, which suggests a fronto-limbic inhibitory mechanism in depersonalization disorder, and has shown how it might relate to the finding of attenuated autonomic responses (Lemche *et al.*, 2007, 2008). The researchers used event-related fMRI and simultaneous skin conductance to compare the neural responses of 9 patients with depersonalization disorder and 12 healthy controls as they viewed pictures of faces showing different intensities of sadness and happinesss. The first important finding of the study was that depersonalized patients showed decreased activity in limbic structures such as the amygdala and hypothalamus, in response to increasingly expressive happy and sad faces. Normal controls, in turn, showed exactly the opposite pattern. The second key finding was that, in the depersonalization patients but not in the controls, neural activity in a region of the dorsolateral prefrontal cortex (BA9) previously implicated in emotional regulation was negatively correlated with autonomic response, hence suggesting an inhibitory role in limbic functioning.

Yet another fMRI study has provided further evidence that, in keeping with their subjective complaints of emotional numbing, patients with depersonalization disorder show abnormalities in the processing of emotionally salient material (Medford *et al.*, 2006). In particular, the authors predicted that, due to emotional numbing, depersonalization disorder sufferers would not show a well-known enhancing effect that emotion has on memory. In particular, it was also expected that patients would not show activation of emotion-related brain regions during the encoding and recognition of emotional words. The authors compared ten depersonalization disorder patients with healthy controls while they performed an emotional memory test. As compared with normal controls, patients with depersonalization did not show activation of emotional processing areas during memory encoding or recognition tasks. As expected, healthy controls were found to activate a number of emotion-relevant brain regions, such as the right amygdaloid complex and hippocampus, as well as the left temporal gyrus and anterior insula; none of these areas were activated in depersonalization patients. In fact, the latter showed no differences in brain activation in response to emotional vs. neutral words.

In summary, fMRI studies on patients with depersonalization disorder suggest that the condition is characterized consistently by reduced activity in emotion-related areas, such as the amygdala and the insula, and by attenuated autonomic responses to arousing emotional stimuli. It has also been found that such neural unresponsiveness seems functionally coupled with abnormally increased activity in prefrontal regions linked to emotional control. How such findings may relate to the phenomenology of depersonalization will be the subject of the next chapter.

Depersonalization and cortisol regulation

Studies looking at the endocrinology of the ACTH–cortisol axis, a crucial component of the stress response system, have yielded conflicting results in patients with depersonalization. One early Russian study found patients with depersonalization disorder to have lower plasma cortisol levels as compared with patients with major depression (Morozova et al., 2000). Similar findings were obtained by related research, which reported low cortisol levels in 8 patients with chronic depersonalization. Interestingly, it was found that cortisol levels reverted back to normal, coinciding with a positive clinical response to naltrexone (Nuller et al., 2001), an opioid antagonist reported to improve depersonalization symptoms (see Chapter 8). Yet another study compared saliva cortisol levels of 13 patients with depersonalization disorder with those of 14 patients with major depression and 13 healthy controls. It was found that the depersonalization group had significantly lower cortisol levels than the depressed patients, but there were no differences with normal controls (Stanton et al., 2001). To complicate matters, however, another study using a dexamethasone challenge found that, as compared with healthy controls, patients with depersonalization disorder had significantly elevated morning plasma cortisol, and were less responsive to the suppressing effects of dexamethasone on cortisol secretion. There was however, no difference between the two groups in 24-hour urinary cortisol excretion. Lastly, a recent study on healthy college students measuring cortisol responses to a stressful cognitive task, found that those scoring higher on the depersonalization subscale of the Dissociative Experiences Scale had greater cortisol responses to stress (Giesbrecht et al., 2007). At the moment it is not clear how to reconcile these conflicting results. It is, however, possible to speculate that intensity of depersonalization and concomitant anxiety may influence cortisol secretion in opposite directions, in a way not unlike that previously found in regards to norepinephrine secretion (Simeon *et al.*, 2003). It is clear that more research is required in this area.

REFERENCES

Ackner, B. (1954). Depersonalisation I. Aetiology and phenomenology. *Journal of Mental Science*, **100**, 838–853.

Beer, J. S., Knight R. T., D'Esposito, M. (2006). Controlling the integration of emotion and cognition.The role of frontal cortex in distinguishing helpful from hurtful emotional information. *Psychological Science*, **17**, 448–453.

Craig, A. D. (2009). How do you feel now? The anterior insula and human awareness. *Nature Reviews Neuroscience*, **10**, 59–70.

Giesbrecht, T., Smeets, T., Merckelbach, H., Jelicic, M. (2007). Depersonalization experiences in undergraduates are related to heightened stress cortisol responses. *Journal of Nervous and Mental Disease*, **195**, 282–287.

Giesbrecht, T., Merckelbach, H., ter Burg, L., Cima, M., Simeon, D. (2008). Acute dissociation predicts rapid habituation of skin conductance responses to aversive auditory probes. *Journal of Traumatic Stress*, **21**, 247–250.

Kelly, D. H. W., Walter, C. J. S. (1968). The relationship between clinical diagnosis and anxiety, assessed by forearm blood flow and other measurements. *British Journal of Psychiatry*, **114**, 611–626.

Lader, M. H., Wing, L. (1966). *Physiological Measures, Sedative Drugs and Morbid Anxiety*. Maudsley Monographs No.14. London: Oxford University Press.

Lemche, E., Surguladze, S. A., Giampietro, V. P. *et al.* (2007). Limbic and prefrontal responses to facial emotion expressions in depersonalization. *Neuroreport*, **18**, 473–477.

Lemche, E., Anilkumar, A., Giampietro, V. P. *et al.* (2008). Cerebral and autonomic responses to emotional facial expressions in depersonalisation disorder. *British Journal of Psychiatry*, **193**, 222–228.

Medford, N. (2006). Emotion and the sense of self: neuroimaging studies in depersonalization disorder. Lecture Presentation, 9th International Conference on Philosophy, Psychiatry and Psychology. Leiden, Netherlands. www.ppp2006.nl/images/Fprog.pdf (p.50).

Medford, N., Brierley, B., Brammer, M., Bullmore, E. T., David, A. S., Phillips, M. L. (2006). Emotional memory in depersonalization disorder: a functional MRI study. *Psychiatry Research*, **148**, 93–102.

Morozova, M. G., Gamper, N. L., Dubinina, E. E., Nuller, I. L., Lebedev, A. V. (2000). High performance liquid chromatography of corticosteroids in patients with depression and depersonalization. *Klinik Laboratory Diagnosis*, **4**, 14–16.

Nuller, Y. L., Morozova, M. G., Kushnir, O. N., Hamper, N. (2001). Effect of naloxone therapy on depersonalization: a pilot study. *Journal of Psychopharmacology*, **15**, 93–95.

Oswald, I. (1959). Experimental studies of rhythm, anxiety and cerebral vigilance. *Journal of Mental Science*, **105**, 269–294.

Phillips, M. L., Medford, N., Senior, C. *et al.* (2001). Depersonalization disorder: thinking without feeling. *Psychiatry Research*, **108**, 145–160.

Quirk, G. J., Beer, J. S. (2006). Prefrontal involvement in the regulation of emotion: convergence of rat and human studies. *Current Opinion in Neurobiology*, 16, 723–727.

Rabavilas, A. D. (1989). Clinical significance of the electrodermal habituation rate in anxiety disorders. *Neuropsychobiology*, 2, 68–71.

Sierra, M., Senior, C., Dalton, J. *et al.* (2002). Autonomic response in depersonalization disorder. *Archives of General Psychiatry*, 59, 833–838.

Sierra, M., Baker, D., Medford, N. *et al.* (2005). Unpacking the depersonalization syndrome: an exploratory factor analysis on the Cambridge Depersonalization Scale. *Psychological Medicine*, 35, 1523–1532.

Sierra, M., Senior, C., Phillips, M. L., David, A. S. (2006). Autonomic response in the perception of disgust and happiness in depersonalization disorder. *Psychiatry Research*, 145, 225–231.

Simeon, D., Guralnik, O., Hazlett, E. A., Spiegel-Cohen, J., Hollander, E., Buchsbaum, M. S. (2000). Feeling unreal: a PET study of depersonalization disorder. *American Journal of Psychiatry*, 157, 1782–1788.

Simeon, D., Guralnik, O., Knutelska, M., Hollander, E., Schmeidler, J. (2001). Hypothalamic–pituitary–adrenal axis dysregulation in depersonalization disorder. *Neuropsychopharmacology*, 25, 793–795.

Simeon, D., Guralnik, O., Knutelska, M., Yehuda, R., Schmeidler, J. (2003). Basal norepinephrine in depersonalization disorder. *Psychiatry Research*, 121, 93–97.

Stanton, B. R., David, A. S., Cleare, A. J. *et al.* (2001). Basal activity of the hypothalamic – pituitary–adrenal axis in patients with depersonalization disorder. *Psychiatry Research*, 104, 85–89.

11

Pulling the threads together

Introduction

As reviewed in the previous chapters, some degree of emotional numbing seems present in the vast majority of patients with depersonalization, with some early writers finding it in 100% of their series (Ackner, 1954; Mayer-Gross, 1935; Roth, 1959; Saperstein, 1949). Such high prevalence suggests that this symptom has particular relevance for the understanding of depersonalization (Sierra and Berrios, 1998). In fact, as reviewed in Chapter 2, some patients do not hesitate to attribute 'unreality feelings' to a lack of emotional feelings which normally colour perception, including that of our own bodies. The idea that 'feelings of reality' might be determined by emotional feelings has been suggested previously in the literature. For example, as early as 1925, MacCurdy wrote: "the feeling of the reality attaching to any idea is proportionate to our emotional interest in it. Loss of the feeling of reality is, then only a manifestation of loss of interest which is, in turn, related to the loss of energy and stimulus susceptibility" (MacCurdy, 1925; p. 126). This idea has found support in neurophysiological and cognitive studies. For example, it has been shown that a reduction in the effect attached to an autobiographical memory can cause it to be experienced as if one had been a detached external observer at the time, rather than a direct participant (Robinson and Swanson, 1993). Similarly, as detailed in Chapter 2, when evoking personal recollections, patients with depersonalization often complain that memories feel as if they really didn't happen to them. In other words, autobiographic memories retain their factual aspect (i.e. their informational load) but seem devoid of the distinct feeling that accompanies the act of remembering (Sharot et al., 2004).

It is worth noticing that lack of 'emotional colouring' might also be related to feelings of 'unreality' regarding one's own body. In this regard, it is perhaps not surprising that those body parts which tend to evoke greater emotional resonance (e.g. face, hands) are the ones most commonly reported as 'feeling unreal' by patients with depersonalization (Shorvon, 1946), as the following case reported by Schilder (1935, p. 139) illustrates:

[Depersonalization] occurs, as I have shown, especially in organs which have previously been of a great erotic significance. I have observed a singer who showed depersonalization concerning speech and concerning the mouth, an organ to which she paid special attention, in herself as well as in others.

The view that 'emotional feelings' may be a core experiential component of perception rather than just a reaction to it, has been a neglected idea in neuropsychology. It is likely, however, that in addition to a pathway of information processing leading to semantic recognition (a 'what is it?' perceptual function), there is a parallel pathway in charge of assigning emotional significance to percepts (Halgren and Marinkovic, 1994). Such an 'emotion colouring' mechanism is likely to be a major contributor to feelings usually described in terms of 'immediacy', 'atmosphere', and 'vividness' (Gloor, 1990). There is evidence suggesting that these two parallel functions take place pre-consciously (Halgren and Marinkovic, 1994), which may explain why, when perception becomes conscious, it is already 'emotionally coloured' (Halgren, 1992; Halgren and Marinkovic, 1994). Neuropsychological evidence is compatible with the view that the cognitive and emotional components of perception are independent of each other. On the one hand, a disruption of perceptual identification with preservation of emotional response has been demonstrated, for example, in subjects with prosopagnosia, who in spite of not being able to consciously recognize pictures of relatives, show evidence of implicit emotional recognition as measured by autonomic responses (Tranel and Damasio, 1985). Similarly, it has been reported that electrical stimulation targeting temporal lobe structures such as the amygdala, often trigger hallucinatory phenomena, which although fragmentary and lacking in perceptual detail are experienced vividly and with a strong feeling of reality and personal relevance. This has been explained in terms of the simultaneous presence of an emotional component that colours the experience (Gloor, 1990; Gloor *et al.*, 1982). On the other hand, a failure to display normal autonomic responses in the face of intact perceptual recognition has been shown in patients with Capgras syndrome (Ellis *et al.*, 1997; Hirstein and Ramachandran, 1997; Brighetti *et al.*, 2007). Thus, while these patients do not experience any problems at identifying relatives, they claim that the person in question does not feel genuine and must be an impostor. The accompanying lack of autonomic responses is revealing in that recent evidence shows them to be instrumental to the conscious experiencing of 'familiarity feelings' (Morris *et al.*, 2008). It has been suggested that the lack of familiarity feelings in Capgras arises from a functional disconnection between face-processing areas in the temporal lobe and the limbic system (Ramachandran and Hirstein, 1997). Similar phenomena have been described in regards to a whole range of objects in addition to people, such as buildings, places and objects (Benson *et al.*, 1976; Abed and Fewtrell, 1990).

Interestingly, patients with depersonalization seem to experience a similar, non-delusional version of this phenomenon. "When I look at my parents I know who they are, but at the same time they feel different, as if they were people I don't really know". In fact, a noted high prevalence of depersonalization in patients with Capgras syndrome or reduplicative paramnesia has been interpreted as suggesting that the latter represents a delusional elaboration of depersonalization experiences (Christodoulou, 1986).

The precise neurobiological structures and mechanisms in charge of assigning emotional significance to percepts, and the ensuing generation of 'emotional colouring' are still far from being understood completely. It is clear, however, that the amygdala plays an important role. To start with, it has been established clearly that the amygdala is crucial for the perception of threat as well as for the integration of fear responses. For example, humans with amygdala lesions show impaired aversive conditioning learning (Bechara *et al.*, 1995; LaBar *et al.*, 1995), seem incapable of recognizing facial expressions of fear (Adolphs *et al.*, 1994; Young *et al.*, 1995 and Calder *et al.*, 1996), voice intonation expressing fear and anger (Scott *et al.*, 1997) and the recognition of sad or scary music (Gosselin *et al.*, 2007). In addition to fear-related functions, the amygdala also seems to have a more generic role in the processing and assignment of emotional significance, as well as playing a modulatory role in cognitive functions such as attention, perception and memory (LeDoux, 2007). For example, neuroimaging studies show activation of the amygdala during the recall of emotionally charged memories (Cahill *et al.*, 1996), and it would seem that such activation contributes to the 'feeling' of remembering (Sharot *et al.*, 2004). Indeed, a reduction in the 'feeling of remembering' accompanying personal recollections has been reported after unilateral medial temporal lobe resection (Noulhiane *et al.*, 2008).

The fact that, in patients with depersonalization, a lack of subjective emotional feelings coexists with adequate emotional motor expressions, gives support to the idea that, in depersonalization, there is a disruption of the process which allows emotions to gain conscious representation, rather than a global dysfunction of emotion processing.

Anterior insula and emotional feelings

Recent research has identified the anterior insula as a crucial cortical region necessary for the experience of emotional feelings (Morris, 2002; Critchley, 2005). Such findings are in keeping with the reduced insula activation found in patients with depersonalization disorder (Phillips *et al.*, 2001).

From an anatomical perspective, the insula seems to be well placed to integrate signals from a variety of sources. It receives visceral, somatosensory, visual, auditory and gustatory inputs, and has extensive reciprocal connections with the amygdala, hypothalamus, cingulate gyrus and orbitofrontal cortex (Mesulam and Mufson, 1985; Höistad and Barbas, 2008). It has been proposed that one of the main functions of the anterior insula would be that of integrating peripheral autonomic responses with central 'cognitive' processing, allowing visceral responses to gain conscious representation in the form of subjective feelings (Morris, 2002). It has been shown, for example, that subjects with a condition known as pure autonomic failure, who are unable to generate autonomic responses, have a reduced capacity to experience conscious feelings, including empathy (Critchley et al., 2004; Chauhan et al., 2008). Furthermore, it has been shown experimentally with fMRI that the ability to experience feelings in response to emotive pictures is related directly to activity in the anterior insula. In particular, it would seem that an inability to become aware of feelings is related to hypoactivity in the anterior insula (Silani et al., 2008). In fact, anterior insula activation has been related to a whole range of emotional feelings such as disgust, sadness, fear, reward experiences, categorization of facial emotional expressions, craving and hunger or satiety states (Morris, 2002). It has also been involved in the experience of socially laden feelings such as the sense of 'fairness' (Moll et al., 2007). Such a vast array of activation correlates suggests that the role of the anterior insula in the generation of feelings is generic rather than specific to any particular emotion. It has indeed been proposed that the anterior insula may be a neural correlate of conscious experience (Craig, 2009).

Posterior insula and 'embodiment' feelings

Experimental neuroimaging studies have identified a network of parietal regions, which seem to play an important role in the generation of embodiment and agency feelings: the inferior parietal cortex, the temporo-parietal junction and the posterior insula. Interestingly, one of the most significant findings of a PET study carried out in patients with depersonalization disorder was that of an abnormally increased activation in the angular gyrus of the right parietal lobe. This finding was particularly underlined by a high positive correlation between parietal activation and subjective feelings of depersonalization (Simeon et al., 2000). An increased activation in the angular gyrus has been observed in patients experiencing a lack of agency feelings regarding movement, or the experience that movements are being controlled by an external agency (Frith et al., 2000; Farrer et al., 2004). As reviewed in Chapter 2, similar subjective experiences are often reported by patients with depersonalization. It is currently believed that the right angular gyrus computes discrepancies between intended action and subsequently experienced movement, allowing any detection of mismatch to be consciously experienced (Farrer et al., 2004, 2008). It is likely that the experience or observation of movements, which do not feel as arising from the self, elicits an attentional orientation response, similar to that elicited by unexpected events.

In addition to the angular gyrus, the posterior insula also has been shown to play a significant role in the integration of different input signals related to self-awareness. For example, it has been shown that decreased activity in this region corresponds with a decreasing feeling of movement control. Thus, subjects with minimal insula activation report such a striking absence of feelings of agency that, when they move, it feels to them that they are watching the movements of another person (Farrer *et al.*, 2002, 2003). In keeping with these findings, studies in stroke patients have shown that lesions to the posterior right insula are associated with lack of ownership feelings regarding the existence or activity of contralateral limbs (Karnath *et al.*, 2005; Baier and Karnath, 2008).

In summary, studies on the neurobiological underpinning of agency feelings have shown that while posterior insula activation correlates with the degree of self-attribution of movement, the angular gyrus in the inferior parietal cortex shows the opposite pattern, so that the lower the sense of agency, the greater the activity in the right inferior parietal lobe (Farrer *et al.*, 2002, 2003, 2008). Another related and partially overlapping parietal region, the temporo-parietal junction, has been shown to play an important role in the experience of embodiment, and both pathology and electrical stimulation of this area can generate out-of-body experiences (Blanke, 2004; De Ridder *et al.*, 2007).

In view of the evidence reviewed so far, it would seem as if there are two distinct neural networks that are relevant to the neurobiology of depersonalization. One first system, relevant to the experience of emotional feelings includes the amygdala, the anterior insula and possibly other limbic-related structures, such as the hypothalamus and the anterior cingulate. The activity of this emotional system is strongly regulated by the prefrontal cortex, and it is suggested that, in depersonalized subjects, abnormal prefrontal regulatory suppression might be responsible for emotional numbing and the related inability to colour experience with feelings. Such a hypothesis is indeed supported by the findings of attenuated autonomic responses, underactive amygdala and anterior insula responses, as well as related increased activation in prefrontal regions (see Chapter 10).

Of the four different symptom domains discussed in Chapter 2, it would seem that three of them, namely 'derealization', 'anomalous subjective recall' and 'emotional numbing' might be related to fronto-limbic suppression.

A second neural network relevant to the experience of embodiment and feelings of agency seems relevant to the understanding of feelings of disembodiment, lack of body ownership and lack of agency feelings (i.e. 'anomalous body experience'), as experienced by patients with depersonalization disorder.

In support of this 'two-neural-network' model, it has been shown that neurological patients with localized lesions affecting either of these two main integrative networks experience depersonalization-like symptoms belonging to the corresponding symptom domain (Sierra *et al.*, 2002).

Cortico-limbic disconnection syndromes and depersonalization

The hypothesis that a disruption in the process which endows perception and cognitive functions with emotional feelings might be related to the experience of depersonalization, predicts that changes in subjective experience resembling those described by depersonalized individuals, should occur following a disconnection between sensory cortical areas and limbic (emotional) structures in charge of processing the emotional significance of percepts.

Sensory–limbic disconnection syndromes have been well characterized in some animals. For example, visually processed stimuli must reach the amygdala of monkeys before they are able to generate emotional responses (Downer, 1961). Research into the sequelae of temporal lobe damage or selective amygdalotomy in humans has mostly focused on cognitive performance or on observable behavioural patterns (Aggleton, 1992). However, some reports suggest changes in subjective experience after temporal lobe lesions. For example, Jacobson (1986) reported depersonalization-like experiences in a patient after bilateral amygdalotomy:

> [The patient] complained of difficulty in describing her own affect, reporting most affects as unfamiliar, strange and vague… [she also experienced] a feeling of being cut off from herself or the world, when she could not think or remember, was associated with micropsia of her hands and feet, and 'remoteness' from other objects which appeared to have normal size (p. 442).

The relevance of this report is uncertain, given the absence of other reported cases. Furthermore, one major problem with cases of fully-fledged depersonalization following brain damage is that its occurrence may be a non-specific response to brain insult (Mayer-Gross, 1935), with the location of lesions playing only an indirect role (Paulig et al., 1998; Lambert et al., 2002). Another problem is that the well-known association between anxiety and depersonalization could confound its association with some neurological diseases. In view of the above difficulties, an alternative approach might be the study of neurological conditions that, although not considered as depersonalization, bear enough phenomenological resemblance to some of its symptoms as to warrant their use as models.

'Visual hypoemotionality' as a neurological model of 'derealization'

Emotional hyporeactivity to visual stimuli (visual hypoemotionality) has been described in some patients with prosopagnosia (an inability to recognize familiar faces) (Bauer, 1982; Habib, 1986). Visual hypoemotionality is believed to be a consequence of a right basal occipitotemporal lesion or bilateral basal occipito-temporal lesions, thought to disconnect visual from temporal–limbic areas (Bauer, 1982). Patients with visual hypoemotionality complain that what they see lacks vividness and emotional colouring, and their descriptions resemble those of patients with derealization:

I loved flowers so much before ... Their charm doesn't enter my mind any more. Looking at the landscape through the window, I see the hills, the trees, the colours, but all those things cannot convey their beauty to me ... Everything looks ordinary, indefinite. I feel indifferent about it. What I lack is feeling (Habib, 1986, p. 578).

Interestingly enough, one of the cases described was found to have attenuated electrodermal responses to emotive pictures (Bauer, 1982). However, in keeping with the visual nature of his complaints, this patient had normal or increased responses to equivalent auditory emotional stimuli (as compared with normal controls).

What follows is a description in some detail of a patient with 'visual hypoemotionality' as a result of bilateral temporoccipital lesions. As with the other published cases, the patient's complaints were indistinguishable from those typical of patients with derealization (Sierra *et al.*, 2002).

A case of visual hypoemotionality

The patient is a 58-year-old man with a high educational level, who sustained a severe head injury and developed bilateral basal temporo-occipital haematomas (see Fig. 11.1). From the onset, it became clear that, in addition to

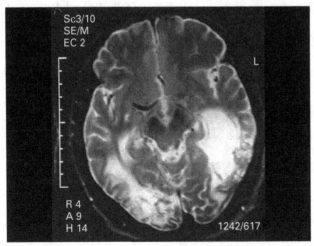

Fig. 11.1. MRI of patient with visual hypoemotionality (see text). Bilateral occipito-temporal lesions are present with a more basal distribution on the right side and left posterior temporal lesion (from Sierra et al., 2002).

prosopagnosia, the patient also described an inability to endow visual perception with emotional feelings (for a full report of neuropsychological findings see Lopera and Ardila, 1992). The following verbatim excerpts from an early interview convey the intensity and ineffable character of this symptom.

Interviewer: "What is it for you to look at flowers, or a landscape?"

Patient: "Flowers to me have lost their essence, I fail to see them as part of nature. They have become almost synthetic, artificial, I seem to lack a kind of knowledge, no, it's not really a knowledge, rather a certain clarity to see nature itself. I fail to see the flower in all its authenticity."

Interviewer: "What about landscapes?"

Patient: "Just as with flowers, there is also an emptiness to landscapes. I cannot appreciate them, I cannot grasp the beauty of nature. I lack a kind of lucidity; a lucidity in my vision that would normally allow me to appreciate it; its colours, the temperature of its colours so to speak. I cannot think of a right word to explain it. I just cannot enjoy that sense of beauty that nature brings."

Interviewer: "Can you tell beautiful from ugly things?"

Patient: "Not in my current state. There is a lack of feeling to what I see. I recently went for holidays to the mountains in California and, whilst I was there, I realized that the snow failed to evoke in me that particular, indefinable feeling of 'snowness'. It rather seemed as something made out of plastic. It did not bring up any feelings even as I walked on it."

As in other reported cases, the complaints of this patient were specific to the visual modality. This suggests that his complaints truly reflected a visuo-limbic disconnection rather than a comorbid depressive state, or even a functional depersonalization episode.

Interviewer: "What about your hearing?"

Patient: "I seem to have become more sensitive to detecting other people's emotions by the tone of their voice. I can tell when they are feeling uneasy. I think this is all due to an increased sensitivity in my hearing."

This auditory 'hyper-emotionality' was confirmed by the patient's relatives. On one occasion, for example, the patient read in the newspaper about the assassination of a famous politician and he claimed not to have experienced any feelings. Moments later, however, upon hearing the same news on the radio, he felt moved to tears. In fact, this pattern proved to be so stable that his family started communicating to him in writing anything potentially upsetting.

This overlap between the complaints of patients with derealization and those with visual hypoemotionality suggests a common underlying mechanism, namely, a disruption of the process by means of which perception becomes emotionally coloured.

Pain asymbolia and depersonalization

Pain asymbolia is yet another example of a cortico-limbic disconnection syndrome in which complaints can be heard resembling those of subjects with depersonalization. First of all, the latter occasionally complain of blunted or distorted pain experience. For example, an early report of a woman with typical depersonalization described her experience as follows: "At present her pain sense is singularly dulled, and when she is pricked she says the effect upon her is as if it were being done to another person, although her tactile sense is preserved" (Sollier, 1907, p. 3); and another patient intimated: "I feel pains in my chest, but they seem to belong to someone else, not to me" (Mayer-Gross, 1934, p. 114).

Some researchers have, in fact, suggested an association between such changes in the experience of pain and the self-mutilatory behaviour seen in some patients with depersonalization (Eckhardt and Hoffmann, 1993). Supporting these observations, controlled psychophysiological studies have found that depersonalized subjects show a considerable rise in the threshold for pain (Moroz et al., 1990; Brovar, 1965). This notwithstanding, close attention to their complaints suggests that some patients have an indifferent attitude towards pain rather than an inability to experience it. Indeed, some psychiatrists likened the experience of pain in depersonalization with that of patients with 'pain asymbolia': "[in depersonalization] there are peculiar modifications in pain sensitivity, perhaps comparable to those that Schilder and Stengel described in relation to their [notion of] asymbolia for pain" (Ey et al., 1947, p. 65). In the latter, neurological condition, patients can feel pain but lack appropriate motor and emotional responses to it (Rubins and Friedman, 1948). Neurobiological accounts of pain asymbolia suggest that insula damage plays a key role in the development of the syndrome by interrupting connections between the somatosensory cortex and the limbic system (Berthier et al., 1988). Such a disconnection would have the effect of rendering pain into an 'emotion-free' experience. More recently researchers carried out an fMRI study to test the effects of a hypnotically induced depersonalization-like state on pain perception. It was found that, in addition to reduced pain experiencing during hypnotic depersonalization, participants had decreased pain-induced activation in somatosensory and emotion-processing areas such as the somatosensory cortex, the insula and the amygdala. Interestingly enough, the latter findings were not observed in control subjects in whom hypnotic relaxation was induced by means of imagery suggestions intended to attenuate pain perception (Röder et al., 2007).

In summary, limbic-disconnection syndromes in which sensory processed stimuli fail to become endowed with emotional significance, exhibit features resembling those seen in depersonalization and support the view that 'feelings of unreality' can be the expression of a mechanism impairing the emotional processing of percepts.

'Hemidepersonalization': asomatognosia as a model for 'anomalous body experience' in depersonalization

The term 'asomatognosia' refers to an alteration of body awareness in which a patient denies ownership of a limb (is unable to recognize the affected limb as his or her own) contralateral to a brain lesion (usually right parietal) (Feinberg, 1990). Early neuropsychiatrists drew attention to its phenomenological similarity with body-related complaints in depersonalization and used the term 'total asomatognosia' when referring to patients with depersonalization (L'hermitte, 1939). Alternatively, other authors have referred to asomatognosia as 'hemidepersonalisation' (Ehrenwald, 1931; Lishman, 1998; Critchley, 1953). As is the case with depersonalization, asomatognosia often retains an 'as if' quality (for example, the feeling as if no left arm and leg existed), and can be intermittent or continuous (Feinberg, 1990; Critchley, 1953).

Patients with asomatognosia can also experience lack of agency feelings (for example, the subjective component of the alien hand syndrome) as a result of the same parietal lesion (Feinberg, 1998). Unlike patients with neglect syndromes or anosognosia, patients with asomatognosia do not show attentional impairments and may not deny any additional deficits (there is commonly a left hemiplegia) (Critchley, 1953). In addition, neglect syndromes and asomatognosia seem to have different neurological substrates (Feinberg, 1990). The following is the case of a patient who developed hemiasomatognosia and depersonalization after a right parietal chronic subdural haematoma.

A 39-year-old woman was taken to casualty after having a clonic simple partial seizure in her left hand, lasting several minutes. There was a history of frequent headaches and vomiting during the previous 15 days. She had no history of epilepsy, migraine or any other neurological or psychiatric condition. Neurological assessment disclosed a left hemiparesis, right oculomotor paresis, and bilateral subhyaloid haemorrhages. A brain computerized tomography (CT) showed a right subdural haematoma in the right parietal lobe and a carotid angiography showed an aneurysm of the right carotid siphon. The haematoma was drained and the aneurysm clipped. She made a satisfactory recovery except for a residual mild left hemiparesis. However, at a follow-up assessment, she complained that the left side of her body felt strange, as if it did not belong to her. Also, on occasions she had the feeling as if her fingers on the right hand had suddenly "dropped off her hand", or as if her limbs had disappeared. These episodes would last a day or two and were not accompanied by tactile numbing or clouding of consciousness. She found these experiences distressing and felt an urge to touch her limbs or pour hot water on them to reassure herself of their existence. In addition, the patient also complained about more body-related depersonalization symptoms in the absence of derealization.

"Sometimes I do not seem to know who I am, I doubt my own existence, I feel like a piece of furniture. I do not feel either a human being or an animal. I can feel the heat and the cold but at the same time it feels very weird. I walk but I just cannot convince myself that I am walking as I have this feeling as if I could not move, as if I was a piece of furniture."

She was not depressed or delusional but seemed slightly anxious. Facial emotional expressions and prosody were preserved.

It is unclear if this more global (i.e. not restricted to one hemibody) depersonalization syndrome was related to the hemiasomatognosia, but her descriptions suggest a close similarity. Indeed, patients with asomatognosia often experience global distortions in body experiencing (Schilder, 1935). Interestingly, an antagonistic relation between 'lack of body ownership feelings' and derealization, was described in patients with full-fledged chronic depersonalization in the absence of any brain damage (Mayer-Gross, 1935; Shorvon, 1946). An association has not been reported in recent series.

A neurobiological model of depersonalization

It has been suggested that ecologically, depersonalization represents a 'hard-wired' response to deal with extreme anxiety, by combining a state of increased alertness with a profound inhibition of the emotional response system by the prefrontal cortex (Sierra and Berrios, 1998). According to this 'fronto-limbic' model of depersonalization, once a threshold of anxiety is reached, the prefrontal cortex will down-regulate emotional processing on the limbic system, leading to both dampened sympathetic output and reduced emotional experiencing (Sierra and Berrios, 1998). Such a pattern of response might have evolved to cope with life-threatening situations in which the individual does not have control over the situation, and the source of danger is not known or cannot be localized in space (e.g. an earthquake). In such circumstances depersonalization will result in the inhibition of non-functional emotional behaviours such as the fight or flight response (the latter is only functional in the case of localizable threats) whilst boosting vigilant attention, allowing a multisensory scanning in search of survival-relevant information. In other words, while the fight or flight response drives the organism to exert control over an externally localized source of danger, by means of overt behaviour, the depersonalization response implements emotional disengagement as its main survival strategy. However, the unaccounted for emergence of the above response in a non-threatening situation would result in an extremely strange experience: namely, the sudden onset of lack of emotional feelings, things looking devoid of emotional colouring, reduced corporal feelings, blunted pain experience, and feelings of mind emptiness. Moreover, the state of vigilant attention in the absence of autonomic arousal might lead to self-observation (Sierra and Berrios, 1998).

An emotion-dampening mechanism might seem counterintuitive, given the importance of anxiety for survival. It is known, however, that under some circumstances extreme anxiety and arousal can have such a disorganizing effect on behaviour that an inability to experience them can have survival value. For example, Damasio (1994) quotes one of his patients with medial prefrontal damage, who, although socially dysfunctional in his everyday life (allegedly, due to an inability to integrate feelings with cognitive processes), was able to outskill the average driver in an incident in which he was able to calmly manoeuvre his car to safety upon skidding on an icy road. Interestingly enough, as reviewed in Chapter 3, depersonalization episodes are frequently triggered under similar life-threatening circumstances (Noyes and Kletti, 1977; Noyes et al., 1977).

Ample evidence suggests that prefrontal regions participate in the monitoring and modulation of emotions, mainly through inhibitory effects on the limbic system (Quirk and Beer, 2006; Delgad et al., 2008; Ochsner and Gross, 2005). The relevance of this mechanism in depersonalization is suggested by findings of increased prefrontal activation, coupled with low limbic activation and attenuated emotional responses, to unpleasant stimuli (Phillips et al., 2001), or emotional facial expressions (Lemche et al., 2007, 2008). Activation of similar prefrontal areas has been obtained when normal subjects attempt to control emotional responses to unpleasant pictures by viewing them with a sense of detachment (Beer et al., 2006). Likewise, other researchers have shown experimentally that implementing a cognitive strategy of 'detachment' attenuated both subjective and physiological measures of anticipatory anxiety for pain in normal volunteers. Using fMRI, these authors found activation in the anterolateral prefrontal cortex as the most likely source of this modulation on anxiety (Kalisch et al., 2005). It is likely that such inhibitory mechanism is mediated to some extent by an opioid-dependent inhibitory action on the amygdala (Eippert et al., 2008), a finding which might explain the reported beneficial effects of opioid antagonists in the treatment of depersonalization disorder (Nuller et al., 2001; Simeon and Knutelska, 2005).

Additional observations hinting at a fronto-limbic inhibitory mechanism in depersonalization come from studies using repetitive transcranial magnetic stimulation (rTMS). One study described the case of a single woman suffering from depersonalization disorder, who was treated with inhibitory 1Hz rTMS to her right prefrontal cortex. After the second day of treatment, the patient reported a dramatic improvement in her symptoms: "I was me again; awake and feeling what's around me. I was looking through freed eyes.

God has reopened my eyes and not just a little." Unfortunately, over the following 2 weeks of treatment, some of her symptoms relapsed. At the completion of the trial, she wrote: "Although things are appearing clearer and more real to me, I still feel as if as though I'm on the outside of myself" (Keenan et al., 1999).

In a different study rTMS was tried on a 25-year-old male with depersonalization disorder characterized by a 7-year history of continuous depersonalization and resistance to pharmacological treatment with SSRI antidepressants (Jiménez-Genchi, 2004). A resting state SPECT revealed moderate hypoperfusion in both temporal lobes, more predominant on the left. The patient received six rTMS sessions (three per week for 2 weeks) over the left dorsolateral prefrontal cortex. Twenty-four hours after the first session, a 15% reduction was observed on depersonalization visual analogue scales. By the end of the six sessions, there was a 28% reduction in the Cambridge Depersonalization Scale (baseline vs. final scores 175–126) and no change in the Beck Depression Inventory. The fact that the above two trials were not controlled for placebo effects precludes any significant conclusions. However, in view of previous poor response to treatment, and the characteristic low placebo response of patients with depersonalization disorder (Sierra et al., 2003; Simeon et al., 2004), such positive response to rTMS is intriguing.

An inhibitory mechanism mediated by the prefrontal cortex on the limbic system might explain some of the experiential aspects of depersonalization. In particular, frontally driven suppression of activity in the amygdala and possibly other structures of the emotional system might lead, via the insula, to a state equivalent to a functional cortico-limbic disconnection that would impair the process by which perceptions and cognitions become coloured emotionally. The latter will result in a 'qualitative change' on subjective conscious experiencing, best described by those affected as 'feelings of unreality'. In view of the evidence that emotional feelings are at least partially determined by an awareness of ongoing body states (Morris, 2002), it is likely that the reduced autonomic output seen in depersonalization is casually related to feelings of reduced emotional colouring (Morris et al., 2008). Although as stated above, fronto-limbic suppression might explain most of the symptoms associated with depersonalization, it is unlikely to account directly for some of the anomalous body experiences described in Chapter 2 (Mula et al., 2007). It is clear, however, that the neural networks supporting body and emotional representation are closely linked. For example, a study using structural neuroimaging on 108 subjects with focal brain lesions found that the perception of intensity of facial emotional expressions required the integrity of somatosensory cortices on the right hemisphere (Adolphs et al., 2000). It is clear that future studies on neurobiological mechanisms of depersonalization need to address the functional relationship between emotion regulation systems and those supporting body experiencing.

REFERENCES

Abed, R. T., Fewtrell, W. D. (1990). Delusional misidentification of familiar inanimate objects. A rare variant of Capgras syndrome. *British Journal of Psychiatry*, **157**, 915–917.

Ackner, B. (1954). Depersonalisation I. Aetiology and phenomenology. *Journal of Mental Science*, **100**, 838–853.

Adolphs, R., Tranel, D., Damasio, H., Damasio, A. (1994). Impaired recognition of emotion in facial expressions following bilateral damage to the human amygdala. *Nature*, **372**, 669–672.

Adolphs, R., Damasio, H., Tranel, D., Cooper, G., Damasio, A. R. (2000). A role for somatosensory cortices in the visual recognition of emotion as revealed by three-dimensional lesion mapping. *The Journal of Neuroscience*, **20**, 2683–2690.

Aggleton, J. P. (1992). The functional effects of amygdala lesions in humans: a comparison with findings from monkeys. In Aggleton, J. P. (ed.). *The Amygdala: Neurobiological Aspects of Emotion, Memory, and Mental Dysfunction*. New York: Wiley-Liss.

Baier, B., Karnath, H. O. (2008). Tight link between our sense of limb ownership and self-awareness of actions. *Stroke*, **39**, 486–488.

Bauer, R. M. (1982). Visual hypoemotionality as a symptom of visual-limbic disconnection in man. *Archives of Neurology*, **39**, 702–708.

Bechara, A., Tranel, D., Damasio, H., Adolphs, R., Rockland, C., Damasio, A. R. (1995). Double dissociation of conditioning and declarative knowledge relative to the amygdala and hippocampus in humans. *Science*, **269**, 1115–1118.

Beer, J. S., Knight, R. T., D'Esposito, M. (2006). Controlling the integration of emotion and cognition: the role of frontal cortex in distinguishing helpful from hurtful emotional information. *Psychological Science*, **17**, 448–453.

Benson, D. F., Gardner, H., Meadows, J. C. (1976). Reduplicative paramnesia. *Neurology*, **26**, 147–151.

Berthier, M., Starkstein, S., Leiguarda, R. (1988). Asymbolia for pain: a sensory-limbic disconnection syndrome. *Annals of Neurology*, **24**, 41–49.

Blanke, O., Landis, T., Spinelli, L., Seeck, M. (2004). Out-of-body experience and autoscopy of neurological origin. *Brain*, **127**, 243–258.

Brighetti, G., Bonifacci, P., Borlimi, R., Ottaviani, C. (2007). "Far from the heart far from the eye": evidence from the Capgras delusion. *Cognitive Neuropsychiatry*, **12**,189–197.

Brovar, A. V. (1965). Skin sensitivity in patients with depersonalization and derealization syndromes. *Voprosie Psikhiatrie Nevropatologie*, **11**, 411–420.

Cahill, L., Haier, R. J., Fallon, J. *et al.* (1996). Amygdala activity at encoding correlated with longterm, free recall of emotional information. *Proceedings of the National Academy of Sciences, USA*, **93**, 8016–8012.

Craig, A. D. (2009). How do you feel now? The anterior insula and human awareness. *Nature Reviews Neuroscience*, **10**, 59–70.

Calder, A. J., Young, A. W., Rowland, D., Perret, D. I., Hodges, J. R., Etcoff, N. L. (1996). Facial emotion recognition after bilateral amygdala damage: differentially severe impairment of fear. *Cognitive Neuropsychology*, **13**, 699–745.

Chauhan, B., Mathias, C. J., Critchley, H. D. (2008). Autonomic contributions to empathy: evidence from patients with primary autonomic failure. *Autonomic Neuroscience*, **140**, 96–100.

Christodoulou, G. N. (1986). Role of depersonalization-derealization phenomena in the delusional misidentification syndromes. *Bibliotheca Psychiatrica*, **164**, 99–104.

Critchley, H. D. (2005). Neural mechanisms of autonomic, affective, and cognitive integration. *Journal of Comparative Neurology*, **493**, 154–166.

Critchley, H. D., Wiens, S., Rothstein, P., Ohman, A., Dolan, R. J. (2004). Neural systems supporting interoceptive awareness. *Nature Neuroscience*, **7**, 189–195.

Critchley, M. (1953). *The Parietal Lobes*. London: Edward Arnold.

Damasio, A. R. (1994). *Descartes' Error: Emotion, Reason, and the Human Brain*. New York: GP Putnam's Sons.

Delgado, M. R., Nearing, K. I., Ledoux, J. E., Phelps, E. A. (2008). Neural circuitry underlying the regulation of conditioned fear and its relation to extinction. *Neuron*, **59**, 829–838.

De Ridder, D., Van Laere, K., Dupont, P., Menovsky, T., Van de Heyning, P. (2007). Visualizing out-of-body experience in the brain. *New England Journal of Medicine*, **357**, 1829–1833.

Downer, J. de C. (1961). Changes in visual gnostic functions and emotional behaviour following unilateral temporal lobe damage in 'split brain' monkey. *Nature*, **191**, 50–51.

Ehrenwald, H. (1931). Anosognosie und Depersonnalisation. Ein Beitrag zur Psychologie der liniksseitig Hemiplegischen. *Nervenarzt*, **4**, 681–688.

Eippert, F., Bingel, U., Schoell, E., Yacubian, J., Büchel, C. (2008). Blockade of endogenous opioid neurotransmission enhances acquisition of conditional fear in humans. *Journal of Neuroscience*, **28**, 5465–5472.

Eckhardt, A., Hoffmann, S. O. (1993). Depersonalisation und Selbstbeschadigung. *Zeitschrift für Psychosomatische Medizin und Psychoanalyse*, **39**, 284–306.

Ellis, H. D., Young, A. W., Quayle, A. H., De Pauw, K. W. (1997). Reduced autonomic responses to faces in Capgras delusion. *Proceedings of the Royal Society London B Biological Sciences*, **264**, 1085–1092.

Ey, H., Ajuriaguerra, J., Hecaen, H. (1947). Troubles de la somatognosie et états de transformation corporelle. In Hermann, C. (eds). *Les rapports de la neurologie et de la psychiatrie. (Problèmes neuro-psychiatriques)*. Actualités Scientifiques et Industrielles, pp. 59–71, Paris.

Farrer, C., Frith, C. D. (2002). Experiencing oneself vs. another person as being the cause of an action: the neural correlates of the experience of agency. *NeuroImage*, **15**, 596–603.

Farrer, C., Franck, N., Georgieff, N., Frith, C. D., Decety, J., Jeannerod, M. (2003). Modulating the experience of agency: a positron emission tomography study. *NeuroImage*, **18**, 324–333.

Farrer, C., Franck, N., Frith, C. D. et al. (2004). Neural correlates of action attribution in schizophrenia. *Psychiatry Research*, **131**, 31–44.

Farrer, C., Frey, S. H., Van Horn, J. D. et al. (2008). The angular gyrus computes action awareness representations. *Cerebral Cortex*, **18**, 254–261.

Feinberg, T. E., Haber, L. D., Leeds, N. E. (1990). Verbal asomatognosia. *Neurology*, **40**, 1391–1394.

Feinberg, T. E., Roane, D. M., Cohen, J. (1998). Partial status epilepticus associated with asomatognosia and alien hand-like behaviors. *Archives of Neurology*, 55, 1574–1576.

Frith, C. D., Blakemore, S. J., Wolpert, D. M. (2000). Abnormalities in the awareness and control of action. *Philosophical Transactions of the Royal Society of London. Series B Biological Sciences*, 355, 1771–1788.

Gloor, P. (1990). Experiential phenomena of temporal lobe epilepsy: facts and hypotheses. *Brain*, 113, 1673–1694.

Gloor, P., Olivier, A., Quesney, L. F., Andermann, F., Horowitz, S. (1982). The role of the limbic system in experiential phenomena of temporal lobe epilepsy. *Annals of Neurology*, 12, 129–144.

Gosselin, N., Peretz, I., Johnsen, E., Adolphs, R. (2007). Amygdala damage impairs emotion recognition from music. *Neuropsychologia*, 45, 236–244.

Habib, M. (1986). Visual hypoemotionality and prosopagnosia associated with right temporal lobe isolation. *Neuropsychologia*, 24, 577–582.

Halgren, E. (1992). Emotional neurophysiology of the amygdala within the context of human cognition. In Aggleton, J. P. (ed). *The Amygdala: Neurobiological Aspects of Emotion, Memory and Mental Dysfunction*, pp. 191–228. New York: Wiley-Liss.

Halgren, E., Marinkovic, K. (1994). Neurophysiological networks integrating human emotions. In Gazzaniga, M., (ed.), *The Cognitive Neurosciences*. pp. 1137–1151. Cambridge, MA: MIT Press.

Hirstein, W., Ramachandran, V. S. (1997). Capgras syndrome: a novel probe for understanding the neural representation of the identity and familiarity of persons. *Proceedings Biological Sciences*, 264, 437–444.

Höistad, M., Barbas, H. (2008). Sequence of information processing for emotions through pathways linking temporal and insular cortices with the amygdala. *Neuroimage*, 40, 1016–1033.

Jacobson, R. (1986). Disorders of facial recognition, social behaviour and affect after combined bilateral amygdalotomy and subcaudate tractotomy – a clinical and experimental study. *Psychological Medicine*, 16, 439–450.

Jiménez-Genchi, A. M. (2004). Repetitive transcranial magnetic stimulation improves depersonalization: a case report. *CNS Spectrum*, 9, 375–376.

Kalisch, R., Wiech, K., Critchley, H. D. *et al.* (2005). Anxiety reduction through detachment: subjective, physiological, and neural effects. *Journal of Cognitive Neuroscience*, 17, 874–883.

Karnath, H. O., Baier, B., Nägele, T. (2005). Awareness of the functioning of one's own limbs mediated by the insular cortex? *Journal of Neuroscience*, 25, 7134–7138.

Keenan, J. P., Freund, S., Pascual-Leone, A. (1999). Repetitive transcranial magnetic stimulation and depersonalization disorder. A case study. *Proceedings and Abstracts of the Eastern Psychological Association*, 70, 78.

LaBar, K. S., LeDoux, J. E., Spencer, D. D., Phelps, E. A. (1995). Impaired fear conditioning following unilateral temporal lobectomy in humans. *Journal of Neuroscience*, 15, 6846–6855.

Lambert, M. V., Sierra, M., Phillips, M. L., David, A. S. (2002). The spectrum of organic depersonalization: a review plus four new cases. *Journal of Neuropsychiatry and Clinical Neuroscience*, 14, 141–154.

LeDoux, J. (2007). The amygdala. *Current Biology*, 17, 868–874.

Lemche, E., Surguladze, S. A., Giampietro, V. P. *et al.* (2007). Limbic and prefrontal responses to facial emotion expressions in depersonalization. *Neuroreport*, 18, 473–477.

Lemche, E., Anilkumar, A., Giampietro, V. P. *et al.* (2008). Cerebral and autonomic responses to emotional facial expressions in depersonalisation disorder. *British Journal of Psychiatry*, 193, 222–228.

Lhermitte, J. (1939). *L'Image de Notre Corps*. Paris: Nouvelle, Revue Critique, 1939.

Lishman, W. A. (1998). *Organic Psychiatry: The Psychological Consequences of Cerebral Disorder*. London: Blackwell.

Lopera, F., Ardila, A. (1992). Prosopamnesia and limbic disconnection syndrome: a case study. *Neuropsychology*, 6, 3–12.

MacCurdy, J. T. (1925). *Psychology of Emotions: Morbid and Normal*. London: Kegan Paul.

Mayer-Gross, W. (1935). On Depersonalisation. *British Journal of Medical Psychology*, 15, 103–122.

Mesulam, M-M., Mufson, E. J. (1985). The insula of Reil in man and monkey. Architectonics, connectivity, and function. In Peters, A., Jones, E. G. (eds.), *Cerebral Cortex*, Vol. 4 pp. 179–226. New York: Plenum.

Moll, J., de Oliveira-Souza, R., Garrido, G. J. (2007). The self as a moral agent: linking the neural bases of social agency and moral sensitivity. *Social Neuroscience*, 2, 336–352.

Moroz, B. T., Nuller, IuL., Ustimova, I. N., Andreev, B. V. (1990). Study of pain sensitivity based on the indicators of electro-odontometry in patients with depersonalization and depressive disorders. *Zhurnal-Nevropatologii-Psikhiatrii-Im-S-S-Korsakova*, 90, 81–82.

Morris, A. L., Cleary, A. M., Still, M. L. (2008). The role of autonomic arousal in feelings of familiarity. *Conscious Cognition*, 17, 1378–1385.

Morris, J. S. (2002). How do you feel? *Trends in Cognitive Sciences*, 6, 317–319.

Mula, M., Pini, S., Cassano, G. B. (2007). The neurobiology and clinical significance of depersonalization in mood and anxiety disorders: a critical reappraisal. *Journal of Affective Disorders*, 99, 91–99.

Noulhiane, M., Piolino, P., Hasboun, D., Clemenceau, S., Baulac, M., Samson, S. (2008). Autonoetic consciousness in autobiographical memories after medial temporal lobe resection. *Behavioural Neurology*, 19, 19–22.

Noyes, R., Kletti, R. (1977). Depersonalisation in response to life threatening danger. *Comprehensive Psychiatry*, 18, 375–384.

Noyes, R., Hoenk, P. R., Kuperman, S., Slymen, D. J. (1977). Depersonalization in accident victims and psychiatric patients. *Journal of Nervous and Mental Disease*, 164, 401–407.

Nuller, Y. L., Morozova, M. G., Kushnir, O. N., Hamper, N. (2001). Effect of naloxone therapy on depersonalization: a pilot study. *Journal of Psychopharmacology*, 15, 93–95.

Ochsner, K. N., Gross, J. J. (2005). The cognitive control of emotion. *Trends in Cognitive Science*, 9, 242–249.

Paulig, M., Böttger, S., Sommer, M., Prosiegel, M. (1998). Depersonalizations-syndrom nach erworbener Hirnschädigung. *Nervenarzt*, **69**, 1100–1106.

Phillips, M. L., Medford, N., Senior, C. *et al.* (2001). Depersonalization disorder: thinking without feeling. *Psychiatry Research*, **108**, 145–160.

Quirk, G. J., Beer, J. S. (2006). Prefrontal involvement in the regulation of emotion: convergence of rat and human studies. *Current Opinion in Neurobiology*, **16**, 723–727.

Robinson, J. A., Swanson, K. L. (1993). Field and observer modes of remembering. *Memory*, **1**, 169–184.

Röder, C. H., Michal, M., Overbeck, G., van de Ven, V. G., Linden, D. E. (2007). Pain response in depersonalization: a functional imaging study using hypnosis in healthy subjects. *Psychotherapy and Psychosomatics*, **76**, 115–121.

Roth, M. (1959). The phobic anxiety-depersonalisation syndrome. *Proceedings of the Royal Society of Medicine*, **52**, 587–595.

Rubins, J. L., Friedman, E. (1948). Asymbolia for pain. *Archives of Neurology and Psychiatry*, **60**, 555–573.

Saperstein, J. L. (1949). Phenomena of depersonalization. *Journal of Nervous and Mental Disease*, **110**, 236–251.

Scott, S. K., Young, A. W., Calder, A. J., Hellawell, D. J., Aggleton, J. P., Johnson, M. (1997). Impaired auditory recognition of fear and anger following bilateral amygdala lesions. *Nature*, **54**, 57.

Schilder, P. (1935). *The Image and Appearance of the Human Body*. London: Kegan Paul.

Sharot, T., Delgado, M. R., Phelps, E. A. (2004). How emotion enhances the feeling of remembering. *Nature Neuroscience*, **7**, 1376–1380.

Shorvon, H. J. (1946). The depersonalisation syndrome. *Proceedings of the Royal Society of Medicine*, **39**, 779–792.

Sierra, M., Berrios, G. E. (1998). Depersonalization: neurobiological perspectives. *Biological Psychiatry*, **44**, 898–908.

Sierra, M., Berrios, G. E. (2001). The phenomenological stability of depersonalization: comparing the old with the new. *Journal Nervous and Mental Disease*, **189**, 629–636.

Sierra, M., Lopera, F., Lambert, M.V., Phillips, M. L., David, A. S. (2002). Separating depersonalisation and derealisation: the relevance of the "lesion method". *Journal of Neurology, Neurosurgery and Psychiatry*, **72**, 530–532.

Sierra, M., Phillips, M. L., Ivin, G., Krystal, J., David, A. S. (2003). A placebo-controlled, cross-over trial of lamotrigine in depersonalization disorder. *Journal of Psychopharmacology*, **17**, 103–105.

Silani, G., Bird, G., Brindley, R., Singer, T., Frith, C., Frith, U. (2008). Levels of emotional awareness and autism: an fMRI study. *Social Neuroscience*, **3**, 97–112.

Simeon, D., Knutelska, M. (2005). An open trial of naltrexone in the treatment of depersonalization disorder. *Journal of Clinical Psychopharmacology*, **25**, 267–270.

Simeon, D., Guralnik, O., Hazlett, E. A., Spiegel-Cohen, J., Hollander, E., Buchsbaum, M. S. (2000). Feeling unreal: a PET study of depersonalization disorder. *American Journal of Psychiatry*, **157**, 1782–1788.

Simeon, D., Guralnik, O., Schmeidler, J., Knutelska, M. (2004). Fluoxetine therapy in depersonalization disorder: randomised controlled trial. *The British Journal of Psychiatry*, **185**, 31–36.

Sollier, P. (1907). On certain coenesthetic disturbances. *Journal of Abnormal Psychology*, **2**, 1–8.

Todorov, A., Duchaine, B. (2008). Reading trustworthiness in faces without recognizing faces. *Cognitive Neuropsychology*, **25**, 395–410.

Tranel, D., Damasio, A. R. (1985). Knowledge without awareness: an autonomic index of facial recognition by prosopagnosics. *Science*, **8**, 1453–1454.

Young, A. W., Aggleton, J. P., Hellawell, D. J., Johnson, M., Broks, P., Hanley, J. R. (1995). Face processing impairments after amygdalotomy. *Brain*, **118**, 15–24.

Appendix: The Cambridge Depersonalization Scale

NAME: _____AGE: ____ SEX: male / female
(please circle as required)
SCHOOLING: primary / secondary / higher (e.g. university)
(please circle as required)

Please Read Instructions Carefully

This questionnaire describes strange and 'funny' experiences that normal people may have in their daily life. We are interested in their: (a) frequency, i.e. how often have you had these experiences *OVER THE LAST 6 MONTHS*, and (b) their approximate duration. For each question, please circle the answers that suit you best. If you are not sure, give your best guess.

1. Out of the blue, I feel strange, as if I were not real or as if I were cut off from the world.

Frequency	**Duration**
0 = *never*	**In general, it lasts**
1 = *rarely*	1 = *few seconds*
2 = *often*	2 = *few minutes*
3 = *very often*	3 = *few hours*
4 = *all the time*	4 = *about a day*
	5 = *more than a day*
	6 = *more than a week*

2. What I see looks 'flat' or 'lifeless', as if I were looking at a picture.

Frequency	**Duration**
0 = *never*	**In general, it lasts**
1 = *rarely*	1 = *few seconds*
2 = *often*	2 = *few minutes*
3 = *very often*	3 = *few hours*
4 = *all the time*	4 = *about a day*
	5 = *more than a day*
	6 = *more than a week*

3. Parts of my body feel as if they didn't belong to me.

Frequency	Duration
0 = *never*	**In general, it lasts**
1 = *rarely*	1 = *few seconds*
2 = *often*	2 = *few minutes*
3 = *very often*	3 = *few hours*
4 = *all the time*	4 = *about a day*
	5 = *more than a day*
	6 = *more than a week*

4. I have found myself ***not being frightened at all*** in situations which normally I would find frightening or distressing.

Frequency	Duration
0 = *never*	**In general, it lasts**
1 = *rarely*	1 = *few seconds*
2 = *often*	2 = *few minutes*
3 = *very often*	3 = *few hours*
4 = *all the time*	4 = *about a day*
	5 = *more than a day*
	6 = *more than a week*

5. My favourite activities are no longer enjoyable.

Frequency	Duration
0 = *never*	**In general, it lasts**
1 = *rarely*	1 = *few seconds*
2 = *often*	2 = *few minutes*
3 = *very often*	3 = *few hours*
4 = *all the time*	4 = *about a day*
	5 = *more than a day*
	6 = *more than a week*

6. Whilst doing something I have the feeling of being a 'detached observer' of myself.

Frequency	Duration
0 = *never*	**In general, it lasts**
1 = *rarely*	1 = *few seconds*
2 = *often*	2 = *few minutes*
3 = *very often*	3 = *few hours*
4 = *all the time*	4 = *about a day*
	5 = *more than a day*
	6 = *more than a week*

7. The flavour of meals no longer gives me a feeling of pleasure or distaste.

Frequency	**Duration**
0 = *never*	**In general, it lasts**
1 = *rarely*	1 = *few seconds*
2 = *often*	2 = *few minutes*
3 = *very often*	3 = *few hours*
4 = *all the time*	4 = *about a day*
	5 = *more than a day*
	6 = *more than a week*

8. My body feels very light, as if it were floating on air.

Frequency	**Duration**
0 = *never*	**In general, it lasts**
1 = *rarely*	1 = *few seconds*
2 = *often*	2 = *few minutes*
3 = *very often*	3 = *few hours*
4 = *all the time*	4 = *about a day*
	5 = *more than a day*
	6 = *more than a week*

9. When I weep or laugh, I do not seem **to feel** any emotions at all.

Frequency	**Duration**
0 = *never*	**In general, it lasts**
1 = *rarely*	1 = *few seconds*
2 = *often*	2 = *few minutes*
3 = *very often*	3 = *few hours*
4 = *all the time*	4 = *about a day*
	5 = *more than a day*
	6 = *more than a week*

10. I have the feeling of **not having any thoughts at all**, so that when I speak it feels as if my words were being uttered by an 'automaton'.

Frequency	**Duration**
0 = *never*	**In general, it lasts**
1 = *rarely*	1 = *few seconds*
2 = *often*	2 = *few minutes*
3 = *very often*	3 = *few hours*
4 = *all the time*	4 = *about a day*
	5 = *more than a day*
	6 = *more than a week*

11. Familiar voices (including my own) sound remote and unreal.

Frequency	Duration
0 = *never*	**In general, it lasts**
1 = *rarely*	1 = *few seconds*
2 = *often*	2 = *few minutes*
3 = *very often*	3 = *few hours*
4 = *all the time*	4 = *about a day*
	5 = *more than a day*
	6 = *more than a week*

12. I have the feeling that my hands or my feet have become larger or smaller.

Frequency	Duration
0 = *never*	**In general, it lasts**
1 = *rarely*	1 = *few seconds*
2 = *often*	2 = *few minutes*
3 = *very often*	3 = *few hours*
4 = *all the time*	4 = *about a day*
	5 = *more than a day*
	6 = *more than a week*

13. My surroundings feel detached or unreal, as if there was a veil between me and the outside world.

Frequency	Duration
0 = *never*	**In general, it lasts**
1 = *rarely*	1 = *few seconds*
2 = *often*	2 = *few minutes*
3 = *very often*	3 = *few hours*
4 = *all the time*	4 = *about a day*
	5 = *more than a day*
	6 = *more than a week*

14. It seems as if things that I have recently done had taken place a long time ago. For example, anything which I have done this morning feels as if it were done weeks ago.

Frequency	Duration
0 = *never*	**In general, it lasts**
1 = *rarely*	1 = *few seconds*
2 = *often*	2 = *few minutes*
3 = *very often*	3 = *few hours*
4 = *all the time*	4 = *about a day*
	5 = *more than a day*
	6 = *more than a week*

15. Whilst fully awake I have 'visions' in which I can *see* myself outside, as if I were looking my image in a mirror.

Frequency	Duration
0 = *never*	**In general, it lasts**
1 = *rarely*	1 = *few seconds*
2 = *often*	2 = *few minutes*
3 = *very often*	3 = *few hours*
4 = *all the time*	4 = *about a day*
	5 = *more than a day*
	6 = *more than a week*

16. I feel detached from memories of things that have happened to me – as if I had not been involved in them.

Frequency	Duration
0 = *never*	**In general, it lasts**
1 = *rarely*	1 = *few seconds*
2 = *often*	2 = *few minutes*
3 = *very often*	3 = *few hours*
4 = *all the time*	4 = *about a day*
	5 = *more than a day*
	6 = *more than a week*

17. When in a new situation, it feels as if I have been through it before.

Frequency	Duration
0 = *never*	**In general, it lasts**
1 = *rarely*	1 = *few seconds*
2 = *often*	2 = *few minutes*
3 = *very often*	3 = *few hours*
4 = *all the time*	4 = *about a day*
	5 = *more than a day*
	6 = *more than a week*

18. Out of the blue, I find myself not feeling any affection towards my family and close friends.

Frequency	Duration
0 = *never*	**In general, it lasts**
1 = *rarely*	1 = *few seconds*
2 = *often*	2 = *few minutes*
3 = *very often*	3 = *few hours*
4 = *all the time*	4 = *about a day*
	5 = *more than a day*
	6 = *more than a week*

19. Objects around me seem to look smaller or further away.

Frequency	Duration
0 = *never*	**In general, it lasts**
1 = *rarely*	1 = *few seconds*
2 = *often*	2 = *few minutes*
3 = *very often*	3 = *few hours*
4 = *all the time*	4 = *about a day*
	5 = *more than a day*
	6 = *more than a week*

20. I cannot feel properly the objects that I touch with my hands, for it feels ***as if it was not me*** who was touching it.

Frequency	Duration
0 = *never*	**In general, it lasts**
1 = *rarely*	1 = *few seconds*
2 = *often*	2 = *few minutes*
3 = *very often*	3 = *few hours*
4 = *all the time*	4 = *about a day*
	5 = *more than a day*
	6 = *more than a week*

21. I do not seem able to picture things in my mind, for example, the face of a close friend or a familiar place.

Frequency	Duration
0 = *never*	**In general, it lasts**
1 = *rarely*	1 = *few seconds*
2 = *often*	2 = *few minutes*
3 = *very often*	3 = *few hours*
4 = *all the time*	4 = *about a day*
	5 = *more than a day*
	6 = *more than a week*

22. When a part of my body hurts, I feel so detached from the pain that if feels as if it was 'somebody else's pain'.

Frequency	Duration
0 = *never*	**In general, it lasts**
1 = *rarely*	1 = *few seconds*
2 = *often*	2 = *few minutes*
3 = *very often*	3 = *few hours*
4 = *all the time*	4 = *about a day*
	5 = *more than a day*
	6 = *more than a week*

23. I have the feeling of being outside my body.

Frequency	Duration
0 = *never*	**In general, it lasts**
1 = *rarely*	1 = *few seconds*
2 = *often*	2 = *few minutes*
3 = *very often*	3 = *few hours*
4 = *all the time*	4 = *about a day*
	5 = *more than a day*
	6 = *more than a week*

24. When I move it doesn't feel as if I was in charge of the movements, so that I feel 'automatic' and mechanical as if I was a 'robot'.

Frequency	Duration
0 = *never*	**In general, it lasts**
1 = *rarely*	1 = *few seconds*
2 = *often*	2 = *few minutes*
3 = *very often*	3 = *few hours*
4 = *all the time*	4 = *about a day*
	5 = *more than a day*
	6 = *more than a week*

25. The smell of things no longer gives me a feeling of pleasure or dislike.

Frequency	Duration
0 = *never*	**In general, it lasts**
1 = *rarely*	1 = *few seconds*
2 = *often*	2 = *few minutes*
3 = *very often*	3 = *few hours*
4 = *all the time*	4 = *about a day*
	5 = *more than a day*
	6 = *more than a week*

26. I feel so detached from my thoughts that they seem to have a 'life' of their own.

Frequency	Duration
0 = *never*	**In general, it lasts**
1 = *rarely*	1 = *few seconds*
2 = *often*	2 = *few minutes*
3 = *very often*	3 = *few hours*
4 = *all the time*	4 = *about a day*
	5 = *more than a day*
	6 = *more than a week*

27. I have to touch myself to make sure that I have a body or a real existence.

Frequency	Duration
0 = *never*	**In general, it lasts**
1 = *rarely*	1 = *few seconds*
2 = *often*	2 = *few minutes*
3 = *very often*	3 = *few hours*
4 = *all the time*	4 = *about a day*
	5 = *more than a day*
	6 = *more than a week*

28. *I seem to have lost* some bodily sensations (e.g. of hunger and thirst) so that when I eat or drink, it feels like an automatic routine.

Frequency	Duration
0 = *never*	**In general, it lasts**
1 = *rarely*	1 = *few seconds*
2 = *often*	2 = *few minutes*
3 = *very often*	3 = *few hours*
4 = *all the time*	4 = *about a day*
	5 = *more than a day*
	6 = *more than a week*

29. Previously familiar places look unfamiliar, as if I had never seen them before.

Frequency	Duration
0 = *never*	**In general, it lasts**
1 = *rarely*	1 = *few seconds*
2 = *often*	2 = *few minutes*
3 = *very often*	3 = *few hours*
4 = *all the time*	4 = *about a day*
	5 = *more than a day*
	6 = *more than a week*

Scoring: The score for each item is obtained by adding up frequency and duration (score range 0–10). A global score is obtained by adding up all item scores (score range 0–290). In the initial validation study a cut-off point of 70 differentiated well patients with depersonalization disorder from those with anxiety disorders and temporal lobe epilepsy (Sierra and Berrios, 2000).

REFERENCE

Sierra, M., Berrios, G. E. (2000). The Cambridge Depersonalization Scale: a new instrument for the measurement of depersonalization. *Psychiatry Research*, **93**, 153–164.

Index

Printed in the United States
By Bookmasters